Missing Words

Missing Words

The Family Handbook on Adult Hearing Loss

Kay Thomsett
Eve Nickerson

Gallaudet University Press
Washington, D.C.

Gallaudet University Press
Washington, DC 20002
© 1993 by Gallaudet University. All rights reserved
Published 1993. Second printing, 1993

Printed in the United States of America

Library of Congress Cataloging-in-Publication Data

Thomsett, Kay, 1952–
    Missing words : the family handbook on adult hearing loss / Kay
Thomsett, Eve Nickerson.
        p.   cm.
    Includes bibliographical references and index.
    ISBN 1-56368-023-8 : $21.95
    1. Deafness—Popular works.   2. Presbycusis—Popular works.
3. Postlingual deafness—Patients—Family relationships.
I. Nickerson, Eve, 1920–   II. Title.
RF291.35.T48.   1993   93-668
617.8—dc20   CIP

The paper used in this publication meets the minimum requirements of
American National Standard for Information Sciences—Permanence of Paper
for Printed Library Materials, ANSI Z39.48-1984. ∞

Contents

Foreword

In 1975, Bill and Eve Nickerson walked into my office in Portland, Oregon. They were accompanied by Dr. Ian Brown, a neurologist, who introduced them to me. On that first visit, Bill was the reason for our meeting. Dr. Brown was kind enough to acquaint me with some of the background of this man who was a Marine combat fighter pilot in World War II and who had suffered trauma that had left him a legacy of chronic pain, which I was asked to help alleviate.

Later that same year, with Bill responding somewhat under treatment, Eve Nickerson also became a patient because she was having a problem with a progressive loss of hearing, which had worsened to the point that her ability to function as a schoolteacher was threatened. Testing revealed that the problem was a progressive bilateral sensorineural (nerve-type) hearing loss. Through the fifteen years since those initial visits, much has happened to Bill and Eve, and our odyssey together has drawn us close as we have struggled together through various problems of life, with some wins and some losses.

Now, in 1993, Eve Nickerson has gone the whole distance of hearing loss—from mild to profound—in both ears. She has resorted to various remedies—from the use of lipreading and hearing aids to a cochlear implant in the right ear that was done in 1985, followed by a revision of that implant in 1988. Dr. F. Owen Black was the surgeon for both implant operations.

Eve was forced to give up her teaching as the burden of communication with her students became overwhelming. Of more critical importance was the forced retreat into a world of growing silence and the challenge of coping with it. To lose the enjoyment of music, the songs of the birds in one's yard on a pleasant morning, easy conversation with friends, the essential professional discussions on either one's business or health, the banter of family gatherings and the laughter of children, all of these taken-for-granted experiences gradually became a major effort to try to reach out and to keep in contact with life.

Fortunately, Eve's family is very supportive. Along each step of the way, through the advances and the setbacks, her family has remained a source of strength and a rallying point from which to press on. Her precious victories have not come without pain, self-examination, frustration, or doubt. Yet, with the help of her husband, her children, and her friends and together with medical advances and new technology and simple old-fashioned caring, Eve has found the inner strength and resources to play the hand that life has dealt her—with courage.

This book, *Missing Words,* could not be more timely. Eve and her youngest daughter, Kay Thomsett, have teamed to present a book packed with practical suggestions and common-sense answers. It provides inspiration and support to all hearing-impaired people, as well as those of us who care for them as professionals or as family or friends, as we all seek better ways to make their lives full, rich, and meaningful by holding open the door to communication.

Donald H. Holden, M.D.
Senior Consulting Otologist
Good Samaritan Hospital and Medical Center
Portland, Oregon

Preface

Missing Words is an unusual book in that it is written from two different, yet complementary, perspectives. When Eve first began to lose her hearing, we searched for books that would help us understand and adjust to the changes that were happening not only to her, but to our entire family. We found none. So we began a journey of learning, adapting, and coping that finally led us to write this book—the book we never found. Our goal is to help other late-deafened adults and their families and friends adjust to the changes caused by hearing loss.

We cover many topics, all related to hearing impairment and its impact on communication and relationships. In part one, Eve writes from her personal experience, explaining the internal and external changes she experienced as her hearing deteriorated. She shares her successes and failures, the coping strategies she and our family developed, and offers hope and encouragement to others who are confronting hearing loss.

Kay writes from two different viewpoints—that of the daughter of a late-deafened adult and that of a student of psycholinguistics. In parts two and three of the book, she presents down-to-earth explanations of how the mind processes information and presents some practical techniques for sharpening mental, social, and communication skills. Kay also discusses how family members can maintain open, loving lines of communication with a relative who has a hearing loss. She presents an honest account of the range of emotions many family members experience, including anger, impatience, and frustration; and she outlines some strategies for improving communication by rearranging the physical environment.

This book is the result of twenty years of learning and coping. In addition, we have asked Donald Holden, M.D., and Dawn Burton Koch, Ph.D., to share their expertise on hearing, hearing loss, and assistive devices. We know that the search for solutions to communication problems will be a lifelong task full of experimentation and of shared joy at the gains and sorrow at the losses. Our wish is that others may learn from our mistakes, share in our successes, and celebrate with us the victories over the missing words.

Kay Thomsett and Eve Nickerson

Missing Words

Part One
A Personal Journey

One

Missing Words

Had I become profoundly deaf at the age of sixteen, my life would have been substantially different. Even in my sixties, my hearing impairment is crucial to my present, my future. But it is not, however, the most momentous event of my life.

Meeting Bill in 1941 ranks higher. So does our marriage, the day after he graduated from naval flight school during World War II. The birth of our children, Twink (Eve) in 1947, Allen in 1948, and Kay (Kathleen) in 1952 were momentous events indeed. Time telescopes, and grandchildren swell the ranks. We look back on other events that recast the contours of our lives—Bill's work, and mine, relatives and friends, sailboat trips—all our experiences weave essential patterns in the fabric of our lives and alter our outlook.

My increasing hearing impairment has changed us, too. In my fifteen-year journey from normal hearing to profound deafness, my self-concept and my life have been transformed. Shifts in relationships between me and Bill, our children, and our friends have, at times, put me at the center of an earthquake, and the tremors have not stopped yet. In retrospect, the beginning of my hearing loss, compensated for by an effective hearing aid, was easy to take in stride.

That first decision to start wearing a hearing aid is often difficult. For two centuries we have stuck eyeglasses on our faces to correct vision impairments, and thought little the less of each other. Yet, wearing a hearing aid often feels like a stigma.

Back in 1972 in Portland, Oregon, I had an early warning system that I was having trouble hearing, and I was compelled to heed it. Teaching the eighth grade in the Portland Public School system, I began to have difficulty understanding the teenage boys who routinely sat in the back of my classrooms. You cannot fool teenagers, they see right through you. For all I could tell, these youngsters might have been spicing up our classroom discussions instead of setting a trap for me. I could not tell the difference and I knew I could not fool them. I needed help, and fast.

I hurried to our ear, nose, and throat (ENT) doctor, Dr. Donald Holden, who confirmed my suspicions. He told me I had a high frequency sensorineural loss, worse in the right ear. "You're lucky," he said. "New aids have just come on the market to help with nerve deafness."

I was embarrassed at the thought of wearing a hearing aid, all too aware of all the jokes about people with a hearing loss. I kept thinking of that old "deaf and dumb" label. In fact, I hoped my hair would cover the aid. It is a battle that we who wear hearing aids go through. Do we not get hearing aids and feel inadequate about ourselves because we cannot understand, or do we get hearing aids and have others think we are inadequate because we need to wear them?

I look back now, years later, from the viewpoint of profound deafness and realize how lucky I was. My hair cannot cover the wires of my cochlear implant processor in my right ear, or the large, over-the-ear hearing aid I now wear in my left ear. But frankly, I would now cart around twice the equipment if it would enable me to hear better.

In my busy classrooms, my new hearing aid was a great help. The earmold fit so comfortably that I could wear it all day. I put it in before going to school and left it in through the family dinner conversations, and all the way to bedtime. I needed to make very few mental adjustments for distortion. Four times lucky. But the luck did not last.

Hearing losses vary. In some people the loss remains fairly constant. A hearing aid that compensates for this loss may carry them through many years. Not for me. My hearing was on an unusually rapid, downhill slide. It was just as well that I could not see into the future. Had I known what was ahead, I would have been frightened and appalled.

Over the next three years, I was forced to adjust my classroom techniques over and over again. I learned to walk rapidly around the classroom during discussions. Standing close to the student who was speaking, I could understand the words. It was more intimate and stimulating to all of us than when I had stood in front of the room.

Although I had never taught by intimidation, during the early years of my teaching career, I was definitely the teacher and they were the students. As my hearing declined, I learned to rely more and more on the students to be adults and to be more responsible for their actions and the climate in the classroom. I had to. They knew that I could no longer distinguish the difference between the intercom buzzer, a cough, or a chair scraping on the floor, so they would tell me when the intercom buzzed or when someone knocked on the door. In fact, I became more and more dependent on my students as my main source of information.

Just as my eighth graders enjoyed adjusting to my needs, so have co-workers, family, friends, and strangers. The most difficult task was learning what I needed from others in order to understand them and then deciding how to ask for it effectively. I had to learn to listen to my husband's suggestions and to not see them as criticism. I had to put them into practice, to struggle with them against my resistance, my frustration, and my fears. It took years of hard work, for both Bill and me.

One day Bill said to me, "You've got to tell people when you don't understand what they've said."

"Okay," I said. I didn't want to, but I tried out a few sentences:

—Excuse me, I missed the subject of your sentence. (That was a bomb. Who remembers what the subject was?)

—Forgive me. I didn't get that. (What didn't I get of all that was said?)

—I'm sorry, I didn't understand what you said at the beginning. (No good. Who remembers the beginning words, after three sentences?)

In the classroom it was easier. I could say, "Repeat that, would you, Dan?" The students all knew my problem, and we were together seven hours a day. It seemed impolite just to say to my family, friends, and strangers, "Repeat that, please?" But I was wrong; it has worked just fine.

Still, misunderstandings were tripping me up. Bill tackled me, trying to break down my barriers. "Eve, when you don't understand what I'm saying, you get the oddest look on your face. I can't tell whether you're upset at me, wondering how to answer me, off in a fog, or just didn't understand what I said. It's confusing and upsetting for me. It must be for others, too. You've got to tell us when you don't understand."

"But won't that be interrupting you in the middle of what you're saying?" I argued back. "You know how much I've always interrupted you, and how you hate it."

"That's true." He grinned. "But there's a difference. I'll know it, and you'll know it, too."

"I can't find an easy way to do it," I responded, and I explained my awkward attempts. Then Bill and I discussed the possible strategies I could use. He came up with two ideas that I hesitatingly agreed to.

"Number one," Bill stressed, "no apologies. They take up time, and you don't need to say you're sorry. Number two: ask for a repeat as soon as you miss a word or a phrase, right at the end of the phrase."

"Won't that throw people off stride? Won't it seem impolite?"

"Not if you smile, and not if they know what your problem is. The quicker, the better."

Haltingly, reluctantly, I began to try. I did not enjoy it, but it did help.

When I retired from teaching school in June 1975, my hearing loss was only a minor factor in the decision that Bill and I made together. When I informed the school supervisors of my decision, they immediately responded by offering me an administrative position, making it quite clear that they were more than willing to find me another job within the school system, a position in which my hearing impairment would not be so troublesome to me. Although school management was supportive, I stuck with my decision to retire. Bill had more work than he could handle, running a real estate office, developing subdivisions, consulting, and starting a manufacturing company. If Bill and I were to remain close, as we both desired, I needed to spend more time with him, rather than in the school system.

I had an additional reason for wanting to be with Bill. Ever since World War II, he had suffered recurring severe head pain. In the late 1960s physicians finally traced it to fractures of his left cheek bones that Bill had sustained while trying to land a shot-up fighter plane, and ran out of gas before he could make Henderson Field on Guadalcanal. He had cartwheeled his Corsair into the jungle, landing sideways on his wing tips to avoid killing himself in a head-on crash. He had crawled out with blood pouring from his nose. The flight surgeon stuffed Bill's nose with cotton and sent him to his tent to get some rest. A few days later he flew another combat mission.

Between 1965 and 1970, surgeons tried three times to reconstruct the damage to relieve his pain. It didn't work. Then the neurologists took over. Night after night, I would lay hot towels on Bill's head, portion out the pain pills, and kneel by our bed to rub his feet. We were getting desperate. Finally in 1975, our neurologist said, "Let's try an ENT once more. Don Holden is tops. If anyone can help you, he can."

So in 1975, there began a collaboration among Dr. Holden, Bill, and me that was to save our sanity and our lives, over and over. Every two weeks, year in and year out, together Bill and I have gone to this large, loving, sympathetic, brilliant man. He held us up in the palms of his big, loving hands.

I began going downtown to Bill's office more and more, familiarizing myself with the office routines, figuring out what I could and could not do—with my limited background in business.

"You could manage our buildings," Bill suggested. "You've paid all the bills and kept the books for a year now."

I was hesitant. "I don't know much about air conditioning units and things like that."

"You can learn, and you can ask me for help. It's the only way you'll feel secure about your future if you have to go on living without me. The more you know, the less afraid you'll be."

At first, managing the two office buildings seemed simple enough. The telephone calls from the on-site building manager were routed to me. I first discussed the problem and then phoned the appropriate contractor—the plumber to unstop a toilet, the heating and air conditioning mechanic to check a frozen fan, or the roofer to fix a leak.

By 1977, as my hearing declined, the telephone calls themselves began to give me trouble. We had by now called in the telephone company to adjust our home telephone system. The technicians had installed loud horns that could be turned on and off, at our convenience, and could reach me all over the house, above the noise of any machine. They also brought us amplifying receivers in all three of our home phones. I unhooked one of the amplifying receivers, took it down to the office, and plugged it into one of the phones. But that was not enough.

The clack of typewriters and the voices of Bill and his colleagues interfered with my ability to understand over the telephone. I learned to turn my hearing aid off and to listen with my better ear. My voice sounded odd in my own ears, but it worked.

I learned to tell Jean Kudlicka, Bill's office manager, what appointments I had each day, so that she could anticipate and help me. I could no longer take messages for her on the phone when she went to lunch or on an errand, as I had previously done. This, along with an increase in office activity, prompted Bill to contract with an answering service to take messages when Jean was not at her desk. This was to prove to be a great boon to us, both then and in later years, as we came to realize that answering services could answer home phones with the same efficiency as they answered them in the office.

As I spent time in Bill's office, he had a chance to watch me in action with strangers. One evening after dinner, he said to me, "You're having a hard time when you meet people, aren't you?"

"Oh, sure, but I expect that."

"You can make it a lot easier for yourself and for them, too, if you tell people, *first thing*, that you have a hearing problem."

"Yes, I know." I knew, but I did not want to do it. In school and with family and friends, everyone knew my problem. Out in the world, I felt embarrassed and inferior whenever I admitted to a hearing loss. I hated the thought of being labeled *handicapped*.

I plucked up my courage, and at times I tried stating, on introducing myself, "I wear hearing aids." When I balked, Bill would take over and say, "This is my wife, Eve. She wears hearing aids." I liked that even less, and told him so.

"I know," Bill said. "It's demeaning. So if you do it, I won't. You're independent, and that's good. You want to handle your problems by yourself. But this is a problem you can't fix all by yourself. And it's not going to get any better. The sooner you get used to saying something, whatever you feel comfortable with, and saying it first thing, the easier it's going to get for you."

Once more, I put my pride in my pocket and got on with it. It boiled down to saying, "I'm hard of hearing." It was quick and effective. I even began to smile whenever I said it. That made others feel better, and I felt better, too. Still, it took two years for me to get used to this and for it to become automatic.

At the same time, I began noticing where I was and what was going on around me when I had trouble unscrambling speech. As a result, Bill and I began choosing restaurants with high backed booths, curtains, and carpets, and no background music. At home and in the office, I pulled chairs closer together and sat with my back to the light.

Fortunately, I had a couple of years of experience and a bit of confidence in the area of building management behind me before I bumped into a *very* sticky problem: a highly inflated and inaccurate heating and air-conditioning maintenance bill. My hearing was still dropping at an alarming rate, and this time I was tempted to duck behind it. Face it, I thought. I had three unhappy choices: pay the bill and feel cheated, ask Bill to take over and admit defeat, or battle it out myself. I chose to battle.

I spent hours going over the small amount of information that the contractor had noted on the stack of invoices mailed to me. There were nine invoices for one month alone. I checked the building manager's daily log where he noted any workmen who came on site. Only four dates coincided with the invoices. Seeking expert help, I contacted a heating and air conditioning contractor we had used in the past. I wrote the contractor a letter, sending along copies of the invoices, and asking him if he could check the work. He did and, a week later, came to our home with his written report. No new motors nor clean filters had been installed, and the new fan was on backwards. Some of the other work may well have been done.

I worked over the fees again, and decided that two-fifths of their original bill was a fair amount to pay for the work the contractors had or had not done.

Now in regard to settlement, I talked with Bill, and his advice, as always, was sound: "Don't go to them. Make them come to you."

Still—yes *still*—hesitant, I replied, "But I can't hear well in your office, and I don't want them in our house." I had not yet learned to *plan ahead*. Luckily, Bill had.

"Tell them to come at noon. Use the front section of the office with the carpet and drapes around you. We'll clear out, unless you want me to stay in the background," he said.

"Yes, please," I said, relieved that I would not be totally alone. "I want to do this myself, but I want to know if I do it badly or well . . . and you may want to jump in."

"I doubt it," Bill grinned. "You may be scared, but you're more formidable than you think you are, especially when you get mad!"

At the appointed hour, the business manager of the firm came, dressed in a neat suit, with one of his technicians.

"I'm hard of hearing," I said as I shook their hands and ushered them to the chairs I had tucked closely together. "You'll have to sit directly across from me, with no table in between, and speak carefully." I had thought that this statement would make me feel less in control, but amazingly, it had the opposite effect. As they shuffled about looking uncomfortable at this unusual seating arrangement, I thought, "Eve: One; Contractor: Zero."

The business manager launched into a technical explanation of the complexities of heating and air conditioning equipment. After a couple of minutes of straining to understand him, I forced myself to relax and listen to the *meaning* behind the words, as well as the *sound* of the words. I realized that my hearing impairment had nothing to do with my not understanding him. He was trying to dazzle and confuse me, the "silly female," with technical jargon. I just sat back.

After he had finished, I opened my file and began to hand him my pages of notes and conclusions, explaining each one. He expressed doubts as to my proof and conclusions.

"Let me see your work sheets," I said. After three years of managing buildings, I knew that every technician fills out a time sheet or work sheet, from which the invoices are written. All my other contractors sent me copies of their work sheets along with their invoices, describing the work done and the time expended.

The manager hemmed and hawed. I showed him examples of my plumbing and roofing contractors' work sheets. "Where are yours?" I asked.

He reached into his briefcase and reluctantly pulled forth some small pages torn from a desk calendar. On the pages were scribbled notations of phone calls. A few noted the name of our building, with limited or no information on time, equipment, or materials.

I looked through them, not believing what I was seeing. "Do you mean to tell me that *this* is all you have to bill me on? Why, on half of them, there isn't even the name or location of the building, much less the time."

"Well, the work was done on your buildings," the manager said, turning to his technician, who nodded his head.

Then I brought out the report of our independent contractor.

"You might want to look at this," I said, as I handed him a copy of the report. I sat and waited, as he read through it.

Finally, he looked up at me and quietly said, "What do you think would be a fair settlement?"

I quoted the price that I thought fair and showed him my pages of notes and figures. He gulped. I handed him a check, already made out. He took it and made a quick recovery. "All right, I accept this. Now, we're overhauling our repair department, so we'll be back to work for you next month."

"No, I don't think so," I replied, as I showed them to the door.

Grinning from ear to ear, I turned toward Bill, who had quietly sat in a far corner the entire time. He grinned back, his eyes full of love for me and pride in my accomplishment, and flashed me a "thumb's up."

Within six months, I was in trouble again. By 1979, my hearing had dropped so much in both ears that I went to Dr. Holden for another evaluation. My audiograms more than confirmed the difficulty I was having. Dr. Holden hugged me sympathetically. I pulled myself together and went back to our local hearing aid dealer to be fitted for aids in both my ears.

Adjusting to wearing two aids is no problem at all for many people. They welcome the increased input. For me, it was confusing, noisy, and stressful. Nothing sounded the way I expected it to. I felt as if I had to learn to interpret the input into my brain all over again.

Bill patiently listened to my descriptions of my struggles. We had learned long ago, in dealing with his pain, that there is a difference between giving important factual information to the people with whom we live—and complaining. If we do not know why our spouse or relative is upset, we may misinterpret the clues as anger directed at us or just plain bad manners. I had encouraged Bill to tell me when he hurt. It helped us both. Now I was benefiting. Still, it took me another two years to adapt to this change in my everyday life.

Group conversations became bewildering. One evening in 1980 when our son Allen (then an emergency room physician at a Coos Bay, Oregon hospital) and his wife Elaine were visiting us, as we sat talking around the dining room table, Dr. Walter Reynolds stopped by the house. Bill had just finished building Walter's new medical clinic, fulfilling the doctor's lifelong dream. He joined us at the table and began talking medicine with Allen.

Walter's voice was very quiet and soft. As the conversation progressed, everyone's voices grew quieter and softer, until I completely lost touch of the conversation and became thoroughly upset.

When Dr. Reynolds left, I said painfully, "You know, I've never realized what mimics people are. You were all talking like Walter

Reynolds, so softly that I couldn't understand a word any of you were saying."

Allen was surprised. "Mom, why didn't you *say* so? I can't *believe* you wouldn't be more assertive!"

Why had I not been, and why was I not all the time? Was I ashamed to speak out, to state my needs? Was I afraid of sounding pushy, autocratic? Were there things I needed to learn how to do? If so, who was to teach me? Where could I go to learn?

In 1981, I could find only one organization to help me: The Portland Center for Hearing and Speech. I attended a short series of large group meetings for hearing-impaired adults (although most of their work at that time was with children). I met Sylvia Tweedle, who taught lipreading (the skill or art of "reading" words or letters as they are shaped by the mouth) and arranged for a few private lessons. It was soon apparent that I was not a "natural" lipreader, as some people are. Perhaps, if I had started sooner when my hearing loss was less extensive, I could have coped better with the hard work that accompanies learning lipreading. As it was, I learned more than I realized from those lessons, but I simply did not have the energy at that point to devote to learning this skill.

It became apparent that Bill and I were going to have to work harder, think more deeply, and find our own ways to change. Even as I struggled to master my damaging emotional reactions and learn the helpful new techniques that Bill and I were working out, my sense of control over my life, both socially and at work, was still slipping, as was my hearing. Each time I felt I had solved one problem, new ones appeared.

By now, I had bought my fourth pair of hearing aids. I could no longer understand speech in noisy surroundings nor in good acoustical surroundings if further than four feet away from an articulate speaker.

Despite these problems, I attended all of Bill's business meetings. We had both become alarmed at his sudden loss of energy and at his symptoms of weakness and dizziness that our doctors could not explain. At the back of both our minds was the thought that I had better learn all I could.

I sat beside Bill in a variety of offices. More and more, I noticed how lighting and acoustics affected what little I was able to pick up from conversation around me. I began to notice the speakers' diction, the shape of their mouths, and the speed with which they talked. Soon, I could tell almost immediately whether a speaker would be intelligible to me. Sometimes picking up just one word would clue me in on a topic, and I would interpret several phrases before losing the thread of the discussion again. I learned to let the words flow around me, watching each speaker's face and not trying to catch every word.

In time, I began to notice gestures: a finger tapping on the desk, a hand agitatedly fiddling with a pencil, a body hunched forward or sitting back relaxed in a chair, a head suddenly shifting. A great many movements, which I might have noted briefly in the past but did not attend to because I was absorbed in the words, suddenly took on increased importance.

Always, after these meetings, Bill repeated for me, in as much detail as possible, what had been said. Then I would add my visual impressions. We found that these impressions often echoed his feelings about what was going on beneath the surface of the words. It was strange, and rather comforting, to find that, with Bill using his ears and I my eyes, we could sharpen our senses to make a fuller picture.

Not only my visual impressions, but the mere fact that I was there sharing the experience with him, became of immense importance to both of us. Never again would I doubt the value of simply being there, wherever that place might be, whether or not I understood a single word of what was being said.

This was brought home to me in full force in 1982.

In January 1982, the cause of Bill's deteriorating health became quite clear.

I woke up in bed at 4:30 a.m. to find him curled up on his left side, his face white and distorted in pain, his hands gripping his chest. Hastily, I placed my hearing aids in my ears, and put my fingers on his wrist. His pulse was wildly erratic—skipping beats, stopping and starting, rushing and slowing down.

I phoned our cardiologist. He was not on call. A colleague answered. I told him that I was hard of hearing and tried to outline our problem. He did not understand me, nor I him. "Never mind." I hung up. My hands were shaking. Fear and helplessness were engulfing me. I had to stop and think.

I then phoned Dr. Holden at his home. His strong voice, distinct and slow, steadied me. "Get him to Good Samaritan Hospital. I'll meet you at the front door. Do you understand me?"

"Yes," I replied, " Oh, thank you!"

I telephoned our older daughter, Twink.

"I'll be waiting for you at Good Sam, Mom."

"Bless you, Twink."

As I pulled up to the hospital, with Bill bent double in the passenger seat, Twink and Dr. Holden, those two strong people, reached out their hands to help us.

Through that long day, Twink and I moved through halls and waiting rooms as doctors, technicians, and laboratory personnel puzzled over Bill's distress. Finally came the ominous directive: "Go to the intensive care waiting room. The chief surgeon will see you there soon."

We found the room and sat down. We watched the small groups of anxious people. At intervals, a doctor in a white coat would walk in, call a name, and sit down with the family to discuss the lifesaving procedures the medical team was going to attempt.

My mind went into high gear. "Twink, I'll never understand what's said in here, with other people talking and the poor lighting," I said. "What am I going to do?"

At that moment, a slim, white-coated man stood in the doorway and called a name. Twink stood up, and the surgeon began walking toward us. I held out my hand, gave him my name, and asked that we move out into the hall. Honesty was important, now. "I won't understand you in there," I said. "I'm deaf."

Twink looked at me, startled. She had not realized that eight years of training and guessing and experimenting with communication just snapped into effect.

His response was immediate. "Sure, but we can do better than this. Come on." We followed him down the hall into a small conference room. As we sat on either side of the table, Dr. Albert Krause closed the door, sat down between us, and laid on the table a sheet of paper covered with a sketch.

"Your husband is in deep trouble. We're watching him carefully. Let me explain to you what we've decided to do."

He was so strong, yet gentle, that I felt no hesitation in saying, "If you speak a little more slowly, and I can see your mouth, I'll be able to understand you, Dr. Krause. May my daughter take notes?"

"Of course. Now, here's the problem."

He turned his sketch around. He had drawn Bill's heart and aorta as it came out of his heart. He talked slowly and carefully, watching me to be sure I understood, and pointing to his drawing as he talked.

"The aorta, which carries oxygenated blood to all parts of the body, has four layers. Up here, where the artery branches off to his left arm, there is a swelling in Bill's aorta, what we call an *aneurysm*. There's a break in all the thick inner layers of the aorta, and blood is flowing through the break. The outermost layer of the aorta is very thin. The pressure of the blood, pumping out from the heart, has caused this layer to balloon out. We're afraid it will break. If it does, he will die of internal bleeding within a few minutes. Why it has not broken yet, we don't know. That's usually what happens. Do you understand me so far?"

"Yes," I nodded. I felt as if every ounce of intelligence and awareness I possessed was totally concentrated on what this man was saying. For half an hour, he carefully explained, step by step, the procedures they would attempt—the Dacron tube and steel rings they hoped to insert in Bill's damaged aorta—and also the danger of losing him, if any step failed. I concentrated on understanding with my eyes and ears, while my mind raced to keep up with him and to look ahead for questions. Twink was writing quickly.

"Have you understood everything I've said?" he asked. I nodded. "You *do* understand, I'm not giving you any odds for his survival."

"Yes," I answered. "We've been there before." I was thinking of the war years, and how many times Bill had faced death and had beaten the odds. Dr. Krause did not understand my remark and looked at me with a puzzled expression.

"I mean," he said, "he may not survive tonight, or tomorrow. And even if we do get him through the surgery, it will be a long fight back. Many patients don't make it through such a long recovery."

"Yes, I really do understand. And I trust you."

I began to think about what I should do until we could see Bill. I should phone my brother and two special friends, Elizabeth Hirsch and our neighbor of thirty-six years Dorothy Hammack. There was no way I could communicate by telephone, however, without an amplified receiver. I walked over to a woman in a blue-and-white, striped uniform.

"Are you all right?" she asked. "Is it your husband?"

"Yes," I said, and then explained the situation. "Do you think there's a telephone with an amplifier anywhere in the hospital that I could use?"

"I'll find out right away."

Within ten minutes, she walked back into the waiting room with a telephone in her hand. She plugged it into a jack and handed it to me. I was overwhelmed with gratitude. That phone stayed there, through all the days that the intensive care unit was our home.

On the seventh day after the operation, Dr. Holden took Bill back to surgery for a tracheotomy because his breathing was faltering. On the eighth day, Dr. Krause took him to surgery again to drain the fluids that had collected in his left lung.

Bill was now conscious, in spite of the threat of death. Each time anyone approached him, he held out his hand and smiled. The chaplain went to his bed each morning to pray, with nurses gathered around him. My every thought was a prayer.

Twink came each day. We lunched in a corner of the cafeteria. When our fears began to turn to tears, she always said, "Let me tell you a joke, Mom." We would laugh, and I learned another lesson from this—the value of shared laughter.

On the fifteenth day, Dr. Holden beamed at me. "I think we're going to make it."

I stood holding Bill's hand, smiling at him. "I love you," I said. "I love you, too," he mouthed, having no voice. In sudden amazement, I realized that not once, through those days, had my lack of hearing been a problem. Everything I had done with Bill had been by touch, by love—that strong, unspoken current that flows between us. If the professionals had anything to tell me, they came close to me and spoke quietly, but distinctly. Most of the unintelligible words spoken around me by the medical team had not been necessary for me to hear. What had been necessary was trust, faith, and love.

When I finally brought Bill home from the hospital, he was bedridden and could do nothing except rest or chat quietly with family and friends. Our personal and business problems still had to be dealt with, and this time I could not go to Bill for help.

Going downtown alone was amazingly different from accompanying Bill when he did all the work. Finding lawyers, accountants, and bankers in unfamiliar office buildings, and then trying to communicate effectively with them, seemed like too high a hurdle for me to jump. Yet, somehow, the long crises we had been through and the friendly helpfulness of everyone at the hospital had strengthened my trust in others and stiffened my own spine.

With each encounter, I refined the techniques Bill had taught me. Each conference became easier, both for me and for the people with whom I was dealing.

By the summer of 1982, Bill was up and about. I began to relax and breathe more easily, instead of constantly wondering whether Bill's repaired aorta was going to give way.

And being human, I began to worry once more about my hearing. I began to use the word *deaf* in referring to myself. Those weeks in the hospital had taken the sting out of that word. It more honestly described where I now found myself. Instinctively, I was trying to strengthen myself to face what I dared not yet admit. I might have to live alone in a world filled with people I could not hear.

With the limitations on his energy and activities, Bill and I were now spending most of our time together. I had ample opportunity to practice the resolutions I had made to communicate better, to listen more intently, not to interrupt him, to watch his mouth, and to touch him more often. We talked and talked, reminiscing about our childhoods, our courtship, the war years, and our children. This sharing of our inner selves, always important to us, now was the center of our lives.

Even as we cherished it, we were losing it. The last vestiges of my hearing declined at an alarming rate. The losses were sudden. I would wake up one morning, put in my hearing aids, start listening to Bill, and dissolve in despair. "I've lost more. I'll never be able to understand you." We both knew that the foundation for the rest of our lives together, however long or short that might be, rested on our deep need to communicate our thoughts and feelings to each other. Bill was as frightened as I was. I was headed for total, inescapable, crippling silence. The loss would be irreparable.

People suggested that we write out messages. We knew that was no answer. Lipreading without sound shows only a fraction of speech. I was not a natural lipreader nor a speechreader, and sign language was no option for us. We did not live in a "signing world," and no one close to us knew sign language.

By 1983, a visit with Dr. Holden confirmed our worst fears. He silently showed me the charts he had drawn of the testing we had just completed. The hearing in my right ear was completely gone. My left ear gave me speech comprehension of only ten percent.

I looked at him with tears in my eyes. He patted my hands. "We all face losses as we grow older, Eve. It's hard, I know." I nodded my head.

As winter's dark rain clouds soaked our spirits that January of 1984, I woke one morning and tucked my hearing aids into my ears.

"Another rainy day," I remarked to Bill.

Immediately, I knew one more tiny thread of sound had slipped away from the precious little I had left. Panic gnawed at my stomach, squeezed my heart, and swamped my head.

Throughout the day, the moment my mind was unoccupied, fear came washing back, like waves. I forced myself to stay busy by giving the house a thorough cleaning. That night I woke suddenly in the dark, the thick absence of all sound pushing against my ears. My heart was beating heavily, and my eyes were wet. The dream I had dreamed was vivid in my mind: I was standing in the middle of our living room. All our loved ones sat around me. Their lips were moving, smiling, talking, and their hands gesturing. No sound reached me. I lifted my arms to touch them, to tell them I was there. My hands hit hard against clear plastic walls. I was inside a big, six-sided box, completely captive and cut off from my family. I could not hear them or reach them. I beat my fists against the walls. No one noticed me. I cried out to them. No sound came to my ears. I yelled, "I'm here! Look at me!" No one looked at me. I sagged against the invisible walls, weeping, weeping.

As I lay in bed totally dazed, words raced through my mind: "You'll manage. You always have. You always will." I said them over and over, like a prayer. I moved closer to Bill in the bed. In his sleep, his long arm reached out and pulled me to him.

In May 1984, Dr. Holden telephoned Bill. "Dr. F. Owen Black, the neuro-otologist I told you about, has permission from the National Institutes of Health and the FDA to perform experimental surgery for cochlear implants at Good Samaritan Medical Center on six patients. Ask Eve if the two of you would like me to recommend her as a research patient. Call me back after you've had a chance to think it over."

Bill repeated to me what Dr. Holden had said. I quickly responded, "Call him back right now and say, *yes.*"

Dr. Holden had assisted Dr. Black with surgery on four patients. If I were accepted, I would be the fifth to be done in Portland. In the articles we had read, all the research patients had been described as adult, deafened after they developed full language skills, and totally without hearing, a state I had not yet reached. I expounded eagerly to Bill all the reasons why I thought I would be good prospect, hoping for this opportunity.

Within a week, Lavina Fowler, Senior Audiologist at Good Samaritan's Neuro-otology Center, telephoned to make an appointment for me. Shivering with anxiety yet cautioning myself to be calm and controlled, I later met for the first time this young woman who was to become my counselor, my friend, my partner, as we worked together to make sense of this peculiar, dimly understood input of electronic stimuli that was to take the place of sound in the human brain.

But first, there were tests, and more tests. Bill was required to be with me throughout the long hours of waiting, working, and questioning. A supportive spouse was important to an implant patient. Bill had more than filled that role. Throughout the exhaustive testing, he always stood nearby and told me how well I had done. The final hurdle came in November 1984. I was hospitalized for three days so that Dr. Black could insert an electrode into my right inner ear. Wires remained attached to my head, bound up by a bandage when not hooked up to machines and computers. I tried one look in the mirror and laughed at my hairdo of rubber-coated wire snakes winding about my head. Medusa, indeed.

My implant surgery finally took place on January 5, 1985. On that dark, rainy morning, Bill and I walked hand in hand from the parking lot to the familiar entrance of Good Samaritan. I squeezed his hand. He squeezed my hand back, knowing I would not understand his speech in the dark.

I was prepared for surgery and lay on my gurney in the waiting room. When I was wheeled into the operating room, I greeted everyone—Lavina Fowler, Dr. Black's nurses, the technicians, and the camera technicians.

I recovered from the surgery quickly, though the hair on the right side of my head had been shaved off. My daughter Kay, who had moved back to Portland with her husband, David Thomsett, came to visit. She admired my hairdo and suggested that I "shave off the other side, leave a center strip of hair down the middle, dye it pink and purple, and you'll be right in style, Mom."

The cochlear implant eased my terror of total isolation. It assured me that I would never live in deadly silence. It also restored my self-esteem as I hoped I would add to the medical research in this area to help others, especially deaf children. My gratitude has been heartfelt and lasting. (See p. 26 for more on cochlear implants.)

In addition, the implant was a dramatic reminder to others of my needs. The sound processor (which resembles a pager) worn at my waist, with its wires running up to the microphone and transmitter above my ear, is a constant visual signal that I am hearing impaired. If people want to talk with me, they are going to have to make an effort.

At first, however, I was stunned by the buzzing, humming, faint tones, and harsh gratings that were supposed to be sound. Even though I had been warned that it would take at least six months to adapt to this foreign input, it was a shock when Bill and I first drove home with my new speech processor.

If Kay or Lavina talked clearly and carefully I could decode speech sounds for a few minutes before becoming stressed and confused. All other speech and all other sounds were meaningless "garbage." I felt like a blind man who, when promised sight, sees only shapes and shadows. Lavina assured me that eventually my brain would reinterpret many real life sounds, even if it might take years, rather than months, for optimum performance.

I asked my friends to read out loud with me, to work on my listening exercises, play the piano, listen to me sing, and laughingly tell me how far off key I was. I kept a daily diary and, with Lavina's guidance, tried anything we could think of to help the process. At the same time, I faced the future with dismay. I realized that communication would always be a deliberate performance with repeated failures. I knew that if I wanted further improvement, it would have to come from me. There was so much I needed to learn, so much farther I needed to travel, if I was going to remain connected to the world. How would I get there? Who was going to teach me? I was still struggling, still deeply discouraged.

On a bleak, rainy Sunday in April 1985, I sat alone at the dining room table, staring at the crossword puzzle. Bill was asleep upstairs, the house quiet.

"Mom?" Kay was standing across from me, concern and love on her face. I had not heard her key in the front door, twelve feet away. "Are you okay?"

I have no memory of what I said. Humans are programmed to forget anguish, depression, and pain. I only know I was in a dark tunnel and saw no light at the end. The hearing in my "hearing-aid ear" had dropped again the day before. At our dinner table that night I had not understood one-tenth of the conversation between Bill, Twink, and Twink's friend Bob Brown.

The cochlear implant was not performing as I had hoped. I had read the warnings that the research team had given me and then parroted them back like a good little student. In my heart, I had expected miracles. I had told my friends that it would take at least six months before my brain made much sense of electronically produced stimuli instead of sound, but I had never dreamed that the noise going into my brain would bear so little resemblance to sound as I remembered it. I felt lost, defeated, and depressed. Tears slipped down my cheeks.

Kay sat down at the table and held my hands. She began to explain, "The brain learns language when you're a baby. Three months to three years old, Mom, that's when you learned to make sense out of babble. Your brain is saying, 'Hey, wait a minute. I did that sixty-two years ago. I'm not going to go through *that* again.' "

"Mom," she continued, "How do you learn? Do you learn when you're upset, angry, or depressed? No. You learn when you're pleased with yourself, when you feel good, when you're successful. Every time you recognize a word or a phrase, pat yourself on the back. You're managing, Mom. Be good to yourself."

"Remember, Mom, 'time, patience, and belief, and the greatest of these is belief.' "

I grinned at her earnest, loving face and rubbed the tears off my cheeks.

"Do something for me, Mom?" Kay asked.

"I'll try." I was wary.

"Make a list."

I smiled. I had lists littering the house: " Letters to Write," "Groceries to Buy," "Garden," "House," "People to Dinner." You name it, I've listed it.

"This is a different kind of list," Kay said. "Take a whole page, not those little scraps that you strew around." We laughed together. "Make columns." She went to my desk, brought back a sheet of typing paper, drew two vertical lines on it, making three columns, and headed each column:

Things I Can Still Do	Things I Can No Longer Do	Things I Might Be Able to Do

I looked at it for a few minutes, resisting the idea. I thought I had been through all that and had come out of it with very mixed emotions. Suddenly, I realized that I had not gotten to the bottom of my feelings about my losses. "I'd better face up to it," I thought.

I began filling in the lists. My grimness vanished, and the humor of it struck me.

I grinned at Kay. "How about a column that says: "Things I Can't Do and Am Glad I Can Finally Get Out Of?' "

Kay laughed, and thumped our clasped hands on the table. "There you go, Mom! Like what?"

"Like having a good excuse to get out of talking to boring people: 'I'm so sorry, but my batteries just this second went dead!' "

I never did get far, writing down those lists. I did not have to. They stay in my head, guiding my everyday life, because Kay's method worked as she had hoped. It made me look at myself, and my life from the outside in. To my amazement and amusement, activities kept shifting from one list to another. As I reached back out to the world, Bill was always behind me, beside me, ahead of me, quietly coaching and encouraging. And I have refined my lists, even added new columns: "Things I Can Still Do, Thank God!"; and "Bad Habits I Never Owned Up To and Am Now Trying to Change." But the list of things I can *still do* is so endless that I often wonder at my continued dips into depression. Yet the daily reminders of loss are real, and I allow myself my grief.

The morning that Kay and I made lists marked the beginning of something new. Over the next two years, Kay would come to Bill and me, at first tentatively, and suggest different ways I might handle the problems I had been encountering.

The first time, I recall, I was sitting in our beautiful, colorful garden, bathed in warm, spring sunshine, and crying. Kay had wandered out in search of me.

"What's wrong?" She sat right next to me and waited.

"It's the words. I can't hear them. I don't know what I'm going to do. I'm missing more and more words, and I can't keep up any more."

"Mom, just what is it that you want?" Kay asked.

"Want?" That didn't make any sense. I wanted to hear. I didn't want to be deaf. What did she mean?

"There are things you can do and can't do," Kay answered. "But what is it that you *want*? Do you want to hear music again? Do you want to understand a TV program without captioning? Just what do you want?"

Well, what did I want? And what could I realistically ask for? When it came right down to it, I could ask for only one thing. "I want to stay connected. I want to stay in touch with the world, at least one-to-one."

"Okay," said Kay. "Then let's start working on that. I've been studying some things I learned about at San Francisco State, and I

Some Suggestions for Family Members

Dr. Donald Holden

One of the most constructive ways that family members and friends can support a hearing-impaired person is to show patience. When we see a blind person in difficulties, we rush to his assistance, guiding him around an obstacle, helping him across the street, or opening a door. Ironically, blindness is highly visible to sighted people. We see and hear the white cane or the guide dog. This is not true with a hearing impairment. We can't see it; we can't hear it. We have no way of knowing that a stranger has a hearing loss or that a hearing-impaired friend is having difficulty understanding the conversation unless that person asks for assistance.

One result of the invisibility of a hearing loss is that normally hearing people tend to be short-tempered with a hard of hearing person. They raise their voices, shout, get upset, and don't like to repeat words. People with normal hearing cannot conceptualize the problems of being hearing impaired, so they have a hard time recognizing the problems that hearing-impaired people face. Patience comes when you realize that a person needs your help.

An excellent form of support that family members in particular can render is to help provide for a hearing-impaired person's safety. Family members must realize that their hearing-impaired relative faces risks that they don't. Hearing-impaired people cannot hear footsteps behind them or someone yelling at them. The family members can help make sure that safety and assistive devices such as flashing lights on telephones, doorbells, and smoke detectors are in good operating order.

They can also alert the hearing-impaired person to possibly dangerous situations such as approaching emergency vehicles, which often can be heard before being seen. Hearing people can locate the source or direction of a sound, and they can relay this information to their hearing-impaired relative. A supportive family says, "We'll try to be your ears, we will listen and alert you."

think I've run across some ideas that may help you. We'll take it one thing at a time, and everyone will help."

And that is just what we did. We all started working on the problem: What can Eve do to stay connected to the world? We delved into areas of study that I did not even know existed, such as psycholinguistics and sociolinguistics. We practiced hand signals to make up for the conversational cues I no longer heard. I studied other people's voices and speech habits, and learned just what I needed to know to understand better. We looked at the problem of how to ask others to meet my needs without my sounding demanding. Gradually, we learned.

"Say, Mom," Kay would say, "I've noticed that you're having a hard time following me when we talk."

"Yes," I would reply. "No matter how hard I listen, I miss more and more words, and then I get so confused I don't understand anything."

"Well," she would start hesitantly, "I might have an idea. Let me tell you about how to use topics and prediction." She went on to explain about how the brain and mind work to create meaning, and how I could sharpen my mental skills to help me better understand spoken communication.

Little by little, the three of us became a team. Kay or Bill, or even I, would notice and define a problem that I was having. Kay would go back to her books and try to find out why I was having that problem and what might help. Then she would come back and explain it to Bill and me. After Bill helped me understand it, I would work on exercising skills that I never knew I had.

It was a "coming together" of so many different paths. It seems now, as I look back on it, like a minor miracle.

Kay had gone to San Francisco State University to major in writing. By accident, she met Dr. William P. Costello, who not only gave her a job and eventually made her the writing coordinator for the university's learning center, but introduced her to psycholinguistics. He guided her studies and encouraged her to pursue a master of arts degree, but much more importantly, sponsored her into his field, giving openly and enthusiastically of his time and knowledge.

It was this knowledge that Kay, in turn, brought back to me. Using everything she had learned about how the mind makes meaning out of language, she began to explore ways to adapt that knowledge to my needs.

It still seems fantastic to me that she would go to one of the few schools that offer advanced course work in this area of linguistics, and meet the one person who both could and would introduce her to the subspecialty that could most benefit me.

Without Bill's love and encouragement, I would never had been able to accept what Kay could teach me. With Bill's help I learned to adjust to my limitations. With Kay's help, I learned to understand my limitations and how to work within and beyond them.

Dr. Black added immeasurably to my confidence in the future. At my request in 1988, he surgically removed my single-channel cochlear implant, which was not working well, and inserted a twenty-two-channel device that increased my ability to recognize sounds.

Even so, every time I sit next to more than one person, most of the conversation will escape me. Of course, I will feel left out. When our exuberant, loving family gathers, telling stories of their lives, laughing at each other's jokes, amused at our grandchildren and their remarks, my heart yearns to be able to hear it all. When Bill has long talks on the phone with our children, I watch his face. I see him smile and laugh, his face alight with love, as he listens to our son, daughter-in-law, and grandchildren. I am filled with longing to reach out and feel connected to these dearly beloved.

Sometimes I feel more than sad. To my great dismay, I find that resentment, even jealousy, creep in unawares. I look at Bill's face, seamed with the deep lines of pain, and then turn these feelings into rejoicing, that he can have this special joy, that it can be his alone.

Long talks with Bill, Kay, and Lavina and with myself, finally moved me into the only possible direction I now must head. There is not, nor ever will be, an easy answer. I shall have to keep facing my losses and counting my gains. I can never stop fighting to find new ways to function when the old ways are gone. I have to keep practicing these new ways—whatever they may be. I will be good to myself, as Kay reminds me, forgive myself my mistakes and discouragements and not ask the impossible, of myself, of others, and of life. I promise myself that I will keep on trying anything that will help me to communicate with those around me.

This book is nothing less, and nothing more, than everything we have learned on our journey. I am still missing words, but I am still connected to the world, and I am still in touch with life.

Cochlear Implants

Cochlear implants are devices designed to provide sound information to people who have profound sensorineural hearing loss in both ears. Implants have been a focus of research for thirty years and now have become an accepted medical treatment for profound hearing impairment in adults and children.

How Cochlear Implants Work

Cochlear implants are designed to help people who have profound sensorineural hearing loss resulting from undeveloped or damaged structures in the inner ear. Those individuals often receive no benefit from conventional hearing aids, and for this reason cochlear implants are designed quite differently from hearing aids. Hearing aids only make sounds louder; these sounds still must be processed by a damaged or nonfunctioning inner ear. Cochlear implants, on the other hand, bypass the damaged inner ear and provide stimulation to the auditory (hearing) nerve directly.

A cochlear implant consists of some externally worn parts and some surgically implanted parts. All implant systems have several basic components, including a **microphone** that is worn over the ear; a **speech processor** that is worn on a belt or in a pocket; a **transmitter/receiver** combination that is held in place by an implanted magnet or by a plug that goes through the skin; and one or more **electrodes** that are placed surgically in the inner ear (cochlea).

The microphone picks up incoming sounds and sends them to the speech processor through a connecting cable. The speech processor encodes the incoming sound into a special signal that is sent to the transmitter. The transmitter/receiver, which may be an across-the-skin magnet/coil combination or a plug that goes through the skin, sends the information across the skin and to the electrodes. The electrodes stimulate the nerve endings in the inner ear. The resulting nerve impulses are sent to the brain, which interprets them as sound.

The sensations provided by cochlear implants are different from normal hearing. Implant recipients must learn to interpret and use the new sounds. It takes time and effort to obtain maximum benefit from the device. Nonetheless, most recipients are happy with the results and feel that their lives are easier because of the implant.

Types of Cochlear Implants

Several cochlear implants currently are available in the United States and Europe. They differ in

1. How the speech processor encodes sound (vocoder or feature extraction);
2. How they send information across the skin (transcutaneous ratio-frequency transmissions or percutaneous plug);
3. How many electrodes are placed in the inner ear (1–22);
4. The type of signal sent to the electrodes (analog or digital); and
5. Whether they are considered approved or experimental by the U.S. Food and Drug Administration.

Implant candidates should determine which implant their doctor provides, how much experience the surgeon has with each device, and whether they want to receive an approved or experimental implant. This information is critical because it may affect the amount of time required for pre- and post-implantation test sessions, the amount an insurance company will reimburse, the type of routine care and maintenance required, the warranty on the implant components, and what customer service is provided by the manufacturer.

Candidates for Cochlear Implants

Cochlear implants can be helpful for many people who have profound hearing loss. However, the implant cannot help everyone who is hearing impaired. In order to be a potential candidate for a cochlear implant, an adult must have the following qualifications:

1. Be 18 years of age or older;
2. Have a profound sensorineural hearing loss in both ears;
3. Have lost hearing after learning oral speech and language;
4. Receive little or no benefit from conventional hearing aids;
5. Have no medical problems that could affect the surgery or use of an implant; and
6. Desire to be a part of the hearing community.

Currently, only one implant system—the Cochlear Mini System 22–is approved by the FDA for adults. The FDA also considers the 22-channel implant safe and effective for use in children (ages 2 to 17) who were born deaf or lost their hearing early in life. (Candidacy for a child is based on different factors than those for an adult.) Several experimental studies are underway to examine the benefit provided by Mini-System 22 in adults who lost their hearing early in life or who have severe hearing loss.

Individuals who think they meet the stated qualifications should contact a physician or medical center that provides cochlear implants. Find an ear surgeon who has received special training in implant surgery. A list of surgeons and medical centers can be obtained from the cochlear implant information hotline (see address below).

Once candidates choose a physician, they undergo a series of medical, audiological, and radiological tests to determine if they might benefit from a cochlear implant. If they meet the requirements and decide to obtain an implant, the surgery is scheduled. During the surgery, the surgeon places the internal parts of the implant system under the skin and in the inner ear in a procedure that lasts two to three hours. The implant recipient can go home twenty-four to forty-eight hours after the surgery.

Four to six weeks later, the individual returns to the medical center so that an audiologist can program the external parts of the cochlear implant system to communicate with the implanted components. It is at this session that the implant recipients first hear the sound sensations provided by the implant. They also learn how to control and adjust the external parts of the system and how to change batteries.

Several additional sessions may be scheduled to refine the programming of the speech processor. Otherwise, an implant user simply must handle the system with care, keep it clean, and replace the batteries periodically. Simple troubleshooting can be done by the recipient or an audiologist. If serious repairs are necessary, they are handled by the medical center or the manufacturer. If new implant components become available in the future, the recipient can discuss updating the system with the physician or audiologist.

For more information on cochlear implants, write or telephone:

Cochlear Implant Information Hotline
61 Inverness Drive East, Suite 200
Englewood, CO 80112
(800) 458-4999 (voice/TT) (outside Colorado)
(303) 790-9010 (voice/TT) (inside Colorado)

—Dawn Burton Koch, Ph.D.
Koch and Associates, Chicago, Illinois

Two

Making the Most of Voices

The suggestions made in the next three chapters may seem commonplace and obvious. You may already be practicing some or all of them. Some of these suggestions are not so automatic or so easy as they appear. It took us a long time to discover them and put them into action.

When a person begins to lose his or her hearing, there is a shift in habits and roles that can unsettle relationships with families, friends, and co-workers. As my hearing kept dropping and I was not able to understand Bill or others unless we were close to each other and face-to-face, I said, "This is my problem, not yours. I'll try not to ask you questions or talk with you unless I can see you." I felt very noble about that offer. Unfortunately, it was not that simple.

Slowly, painfully, we all eventually made a habit of the following "do's and don't's."

Watch the Person Who Is Talking

People who wear a hearing aid have a tendency to turn the ear with the hearing aid toward the speaker. This is also true for people who are more hard of hearing in one ear or the other. They will almost always cock their good ear toward the speaker. They may gain a little more sound but lose a large amount of visual information.

Even a person who can hear perfectly will tend to miss many more words if not looking directly at the speaker. This is doubly true for people who have suffered a hearing loss. If listeners are not focused clearly on the speaker's facial features, they may miss such cues as eyebrows raised to denote a question, a widening of the eyes to show surprise, a little smile for humor, or a tiny frown of concentration.

Also, many of us lipread far more than we realize. When I learned to look at the mouths of people talking to me, instead of gazing into their eyes (and it took me a long time to change this habit), I found that I could tell the difference between some of those indistinguishable speech sounds that I was misinterpreting. I could see a *b, p, m, ow, oh, you, v* quite easily. Gradually, I became more adept at lipreading or, technically speaking, speechreading, out of sheer necessity, even though the concentration required is tiring for me. Some people are "natural" lipreaders. I am not. Yet, practice with lipreading tapes (see Reference Section) and constant attention to people's mouths continue to improve my skills.

The other side of the coin is that people tend to imitate behavior. If I am looking squarely at the speaker, it is much more likely that the speaker will look squarely back at me and not talk to a lamp or a chair. And since one barrier to good communication is not getting all the signals possible, both visual and aural, I am overcoming a pretty big problem.

Of course, sometimes all the good examples in the world will not get speakers to look directly at me or take their hands away from their mouths when speaking, but I found that I cannot expect people to follow my directions if I do not. So if, after I have set a mighty good example, the speakers still do not look directly at me, or if they cover their mouths, or if they are in the habit of turning their heads away halfway through a sentence, then I gently remind them that I need to see their whole face clearly when they are talking to me.

Speak as Clearly as You Can

I am constantly amazed at how long it took me to discover this simple idea: If I want others to enunciate carefully to me, I have to set the example. Yet, when I finally did see the light, I was stunned at how difficult it was and at how much I was asking others to do for me. And, I must admit, I was not only expecting others to do this, but I was becoming angry, frustrated, and upset at them when they did not.

Changing Speech Habits

Dr. Donald Holden

Speech habits can be very difficult to change. We become used to certain behaviors over a long period of time and those behaviors become a part of us, fixed and unchanging. Children find it much easier to change their habits simply because they haven't had them that long. They are more flexible, adaptable, and open, not fixed in a particular attitude. As we grow older we lose our ability to adapt to new circumstances. When trying to change our speech habits to accommodate a hearing-impaired person, we must work very hard indeed. We also must constantly remind ourselves that we hold the advantage and should be responsive to making the adjustment.

I am a fast talker, by nature and circumstance. I grew up in Brooklyn, New York, where life sped along at a fast pace. The youngest of five noisy children, I learned to get my words in fast, interrupting and hurrying, skipping and slurring.

Learning to pronounce every vowel and consonant, to pause between phrases, and to order my thoughts into logical sequence, all were, and still are, difficult for me. I constantly remind myself of this when I become impatient and upset with others who forget to be careful on my behalf. Now I try to remember that the more difficulty that I have in understanding someone else, the more carefully I must speak.

The problem that arises with this strategy is that as people lose more and more of their hearing, they do not enunciate as well as they should. This is natural and understandable since, in many cases, they cannot hear exactly what they are saying. For example, if they cannot hear the *th* at the end of a word they say, then they cannot correct themselves. But I get around this problem by consciously trying to pronounce words as best I can. I sometimes pretend that I am an actor trained to speak very clearly, and I attempt to pronounce every letter or sound combination.

By the same token, I can, to some extent, adjust my speech to the pace I need from others. For example, if my friends have a habit of talking too quickly and running all the words together, I try slowing my own pace to set an example of what I want my friends to do.

Consciously pronounce your words well, and the odds are others will begin to pronounce theirs better. And they will also begin to match your pace.

This approach does not always work as well as it might. Sometimes you will have to remind people gently that they need to look at you, to slow down ("A little more slowly, please?"), to pronounce their words more clearly ("Can you say that more carefully, please?"), or to pause between phrases ("Can you pause a second . . . between phrases . . . like this . . . so my brain . . . can catch up? Great! Thanks!").

But just reminding them is not enough. You have to take the initiative and set the example. If you do not care enough to do your best, why should they?

Do Not Be Afraid to Give Directions

There is a difference between helping people communicate with you and criticizing them. If you are doing your best to be a good example, then you have every right to ask others to try to accommodate you. Often others will talk too quickly or too slowly, too softly or too loudly, because they do not know exactly what level is best for you. They may not be aware of your hearing loss, or they know but do not understand what to do to help you understand them. If you smile pleasantly while you inform them, they will be surprisingly grateful and relieved.

Getting around this problem involves a couple of steps: First, you have to decide how loudly you need people to talk, whether you hear high or low pitched voices best, and how quickly others should talk. This will take some experimentation on your part. Let's examine each factor.

Loudness

Loudness is a very sensitive issue. People who talk to me more loudly think that they are being considerate and are doing the right thing. Yes, I sometimes do need a higher volume than a person with normal hearing would need, but not in all circumstances.

For some people with a hearing loss, volume is not the issue at all. Sensitive hearing aids will give them the volume they need automatically, but the speaker does not know that. Be careful of people's feelings when they speak too loudly. If you just say, "Not so loud," you could inadvertently offend someone who was really trying to meet your needs. It is as if you were saying, "You're a poor communicator." Actually, they are trying to accommodate you, which probably means that they will respond positively if given a little feedback. This is one reason why it is so important for you to understand exactly what you need others to do for you.

When people talk more loudly, they usually raise the pitch of their voice, which is something you will need to caution them about. When you want a person to speak more loudly, make your directions clear and concise: "Your deep (or slow or well-pitched) voice will be easy for me to hear if you could just speak a little more softly."

Everyone has a comfort range for loudness, and you need to find what yours is. Listen very carefully and try to decide whether you are straining to hear the speakers. If so, you will want to have them speak up. On the other hand, if you feel like turning down your hearing aid or backing up about six feet every time certain people come by, you will have to ask them to lower their voice a tad, while thanking them for trying to help you.

Pitch

People often confuse pitch and loudness, but they are really two different things. Pitch is how high or low, musically, a person talks. For example, the lowest pitch is bass, which is very low indeed. The next is baritone, and the middle range is tenor. Women with low voices are sometimes tenors, and many men with higher voices are also tenors. Men usually pitch their voices naturally at bass, baritone, or tenor. Lastly, the two higher pitches are mezzo-soprano and soprano. Mezzo-soprano is just above tenor, while soprano is the highest. Women and young children are usually mezzo-soprano or soprano. (Although there are more than five pitches, these five are all you really need to help you discover what pitches you hear best.)

Hearing aids make you more conscious of differences in loudness and pitch. Just as a microphone both harshens and muffles a speaker's voice, so will hearing aids. Some voices may be more comfortable and easier for you to understand than others. A man's medium-low voice can be particularly restful, while a child's high, soprano voice can be uncomfortably shrill.

Your task is to decide which pitch you hear better, and this is not all that easy. Remember, loudness has nothing to do with pitch. You need to listen beyond the loudness and to decide whether or not you usually have trouble hearing men with deep, soft voices (bass) or children with high voices (soprano). By paying attention to people you do hear well and those you do not, you can begin to understand which pitch is best for you. Once you know that, you can then ask your friends to adjust their voices, as much as they comfortably can, either by speaking more closely to the pitch you hear best or by speaking more loudly and enunciating better to make up for the fact that you cannot hear that particular voice pitch well.

Speed

The quickness with which others talk can be a complicated issue in terms of understanding a conversation. When people talk so quickly that their words run together, of course I ask them to slow down. But, I also need to ask them to slow down without making speech unnatural. Slowing down speech means that the little pauses between words need to be slightly longer, and the longer pauses, such as those between phrases and clauses or even between sentences, need to be longer still. When people put the same amount of pause between every word, talking (pause) like (pause) a (pause) robot, then the cadence, or rhythm, of speech is lost, and this makes it much harder to understand. If you say, "I can under-stand you better (pause) if you pause a little bit (pause) between phrases (pause) the way I am doing now," you will have shown them exactly how to speak. After all, you are trying to get all the infor-mation you possibly can, and speech rhythm provides clues to meaning, too (see chapter 7).

Pronunciation

Sloppy speech habits are a major cause of misunderstandings in daily conversations. They are also the number-one cause of frus-tration for hard of hearing listeners. But again, we cannot expect others to change their ways if we don't first change ours.

I try to be more aware of my speech by pronouncing each word distinctly. This can be more difficult than you expect. For example, when is the last time you pronounced, really said the *t* in the word *not*? Like me, you probably say the *n* and *o* and then just touch your tongue to the roof of your mouth for the *t*. Well, the good news is you still do not have to say the *t* in *not*. But the bad news is that you need to acknowledge its existence with a slight pause before saying the next word. What we are aiming for is to be more careful about how we form words and to shape the words more deliberately, keeping in mind their spellings, their beginnings, and especially their endings.

The aim of articulating carefully is two-fold. First, as my hearing deteriorated, I found I could no longer clearly hear what I was saying. My already hasty speech patterns became more and more sloppy. As my speech deteriorated, so did the speech of others, and this is the second point. We want others to pronounce their words carefully, so we have to show them what to do by example, as best as we can.

Putting It All Together

All the things we talked about work together to create clear, understandable speech. Loudness, pitch, speed, and pronunciation all get mixed together when we talk, and it can be difficult to separate them out, especially when sometimes all I hear is muffled, indistinguishable sound. Try this, just for a minute. Instead of thinking of speech as words we can read aloud, think of it as sound, and write down what you hear.

For example, my daughter Twink once said to me, "Ino wha-dims a-poz ta-do . . . bu'do-ing-it sanather-madder."

"Ah," you say. "The poor dear can't speak English." Yes she can! And what's more, I understood every word. What she said was, "I know what I'm supposed to do, but doing it's another matter."

What we are after here is not to produce every single letter and every single pause. Rather, we are trying to improve, so we understand something like this, "Ino what I'm sa-posed ta-do . . . but do-ing it-s-a nother mat-er."

Please notice that not all the letters in the last example are the same as in the written version. We do not want to corrupt our speech or have others corrupt theirs. We just need to try to do better, as with the *t* in *matter*. And we want to help others do better, too.

The Speech Rating Chart

The speech rating chart (see p. 39) is a guide to identify the voices you hear best. Kay helped me devise this chart because I could not understand why I distinguished some people's voices, while others baffled me. It will help you to know at the beginning of a conversation whether or not you are likely to have trouble with a particular speaker's voice. This is important, for several reasons: If you know immediately that a person's voice is going to be too high or low, too soft or loud, then you will know what to ask for quickly—without losing any valuable information. The other reason is that you may need to delay the conversation or to move to a quieter spot. This is best done right at the beginning. If you wait too long to suggest that you find a quieter spot, then you will have to interrupt the speaker in the middle of the conversation. More importantly, you may have already missed so much that you will need to have the speaker repeat what was said or spend the first few moments just trying to catch up, both of which can be frustrating and confusing.

Identifying the voices you hear best is really very easy. All you need to do is fill in the chart. Your friends, business acquaintances, neighbors, and children can all provide a wonderful source of information. To obtain best results, vary the ages of the people you put in your chart and use an equal number of men and women.

Speaker's Name

Fill in the person's name.

Pitch

Identify the pitch that you feel best corresponds with the pitch of a person's voice and enter it on the chart. You will probably find that one particular pitch is best for you, but you cannot ask everyone to speak at that pitch. They can't. You can ask them, however, to talk a bit higher or lower within their range. Most people have a speaking range of about eight whole notes, or one octave (although trained people, such as actors or singers, have a larger range). If your best hearing range is the same as mine, which is

Speech Rating Chart

Speaker's Name:

1. Pitch	2. Loudness	3. Speed	4. Pronun-ciation	5. Overall Rating

Speaker's Name:

1. Pitch	2. Loudness	3. Speed	4. Pronun-ciation	5. Overall Rating

Speaker's Name:

1. Pitch	2. Loudness	3. Speed	4. Pronun-ciation	5. Overall Rating

Speaker's Name:

1. Pitch	2. Loudness	3. Speed	4. Pronun-ciation	5. Overall Rating

Speaker's Name:

1. Pitch	2. Loudness	3. Speed	4. Pronun-ciation	5. Overall Rating

Speaker's Name:

1. Pitch	2. Loudness	3. Speed	4. Pronun-ciation	5. Overall Rating

tenor, and you have a loved one or friend who is a mezzo-soprano, then that individual will never truly speak in your best hearing range. However, he or she can lower his or her voice as much as possible, and you will notice a big difference right away. As a reminder, the five pitches we described are listed below.

1. **Soprano**—The highest pitch. Many children and women fall in this group.
2. **Mezzo-Soprano**—The second highest pitch. Teenage boys and many women fall into this category.
3. **Tenor**—The middle range. Women with low voices or men with higher male voices fall in this range.
4. **Baritone**—The middle–low pitch. Usually, only men fall into this category.
5. **Bass**—The very lowest men's voice pitch.

Loudness

In this box you rate how loud the speaker's voice sounded to you. The speaker may not be actually shouting or whispering, but it can sound like that to you. Gauge the loudness of each of the speakers *as you hear it.*

1. If the speaker is whispering, then enter a *1* in the box.
2. If the speaker is shouting, then enter a *2.*
3. If the speaker is too soft, then enter a *3.*
4. If the speaker is loud, then enter a *4.*
5. If the speaker is just right, then enter a *5.*

Speed

The rate at which a speaker talks will affect your ability to understand what that speaker is saying. Use the following scale to identify the speed of speech.

1. If the speaker is supersonic, then enter a *1* in the box.
2. If the speaker is way too fast, then enter a *2.*

3. If the speaker is fast, then enter a *3*.
4. If the speaker is too slow, then enter a *4*.
5. If the speaker is just right, then enter a *5*.

Pronunciation

Crisp articulation can make up for a lot of problems in other areas. My daughter Kay's natural speaking range is not the same as my best hearing range, yet I understand her better than almost anyone else because she pronounces her words very carefully. Rate speakers on how clearly they pronounce their words.

1. If the speaker talks without moving his or her mouth, then enter a *1* in the box.
2. If the speaker is mushy, then enter a *2*.
3. If the speaker is okay, then enter a *3*.
4. If the speaker is good, then enter a *4*.
5. If the speaker is crisp and clear, then enter a *5*.

Overall Rating

In this box you summarize your general impression of each particular speaker. If the speaker was very easy to understand, or even helped you forget your impairment for a while, then you would give such a person an overall rating of 5. On the other hand, if the speaker's pitch was too low, the pace was rushed, the words were slurred together, and you could just barely understand anything, then that person would rate a 1. Be honest in your assessments. Remember, this chart is supposed to help you.

1. If the speaker was unintelligible, then enter a *1* in the box.
2. If the speaker was almost understandable, enter a *2*.
3. If the speaker was understandable, enter a *3*.
4. If the speaker was clear, enter a *4*.
5. If the speaker was excellent, enter a *5*.

The Results

When you have the chart all filled in with a number of different people and their speech patterns, then take a good look at the

Overall Rating box. Every person that got a 4 or 5 will be giving you clues to what you will need to ask of all those who did not score as high. Look at the top-scoring voices: What pitch are they? Listen carefully to them the next time you see them. Ideally, listen to them when they are talking to someone else so you do not have to keep track of the conversation, then you can focus all your attention on their voice qualities.

When you are able to determine just what those people are doing that helps you so much, then you will know exactly what to ask from others. For example, if one of your speakers has the wrong pitch, speaks too softly and too slowly, but has excellent pronunciation skills, you may have given that person a 4 because good pronunciation is so vital. But if you are going to get into a prolonged conversation with this person, then you might want to have him or her speak more loudly, too.

Loudness is usually the easiest voice quality for people to adjust. Speed is the next easiest, while pronunciation is difficult to change, and pitch is the most difficult voice quality to change. If your family members and close friends or business associates can make just a few changes (at your direction), you will find that you hear them much better. But you will need to forgive them when they tire or forget. And you will probably need to remind them again and again. So it really helps if you know exactly what you are asking for and remain totally consistent in what you ask. And of course, the last piece of the puzzle is that others will be much more willing to change their speech habits if your speech reflects exactly what you are asking from them.

Three

You and Your Environment

When a hearing loss threatens your ability to function in your home, your workplace, and the world around you, the name of the game is *change*. Change whatever you can in your environment to make speech more easily understood. Then change how you reach out to your environment through new techniques and new technology, with telephones, television, and travel. In this chapter we suggest just a few ways you, your family, and your friends can change your surroundings to improve communication.

Above all, do not give up! Don't give up your job for a less desirable one unless you have tried every possible ploy and sought all possible advice from the people with whom you work and the organizations available to help you (see the Reference Section). Don't give up on your activities, and on your interaction with your friends, your co-workers, and especially your family.

Lighting

We start with this topic because lighting can be controlled easily, and you can see positive results right away.

Lighting that is inadequate or from the wrong direction can adversely affect your ability to understand a speaker. In order to get all the information possible, you must be in a well-lit room. The light should shine directly at the speaker and away from your own eyes. Remember, the room needs to be bright; one or two table lamps are not enough.

Adjusting the lighting and seating arrangements in your home can vastly improve communication. For example, if you have a wall with a window in it, do not put your sofa against that wall. While windows provide wonderful light, they also backlight anyone sitting in front of them, making it difficult for you to see the speaker's mouth. If you can, move the couch at a ninety degree angle to the window, or better yet, to face the window. Arrange the rest of the furniture to face the other available light sources. If the living room or den arrangement will not allow you to do this, then escort your guests to chairs facing the window and you sit on the couch.

At night or in dark rooms with few windows, one easy and relatively inexpensive solution is track lighting. These gentle spot lights on a metal track can be moved along the track and adjusted to catch just about any corner of the room. Track lighting that is affixed on two walls and carefully adjusted can make the room come alive for you.

Another nice thing about modern track lighting is that it can either be wired into a wall or hung with a cord that plugs into an existing outlet. (This is especially good for renters and people who move often). The portable track lights are easy to install: just put up the track according to the directions, snap in the lights, and plug the track in. Built-in track lighting may require professional installation, but it can give you more flexibility in lighting long rooms and is less visible.

You can also purchase individual spots that swivel, if you only need to light one or two particular areas. These can be either portable or built-in, depending on what suits you. Any good lighting supply store will have a variety of track and spot lights on hand and can assist you in making the best selection.

Furniture

From my informal study of living rooms, I can see that people do not like to sit too close to each other. In some cases, I found as much as a seven-foot distance between the couch and the chair facing it. This kind of arrangement is not good for conversation, especially if any of the listeners are hard of hearing.

If your furniture is arranged with four feet or more between the chairs and the couch, you can pull a chair forward and put yourself in the best position to hear the speaker. If another person is added to the group, you can then quickly move your chair to include the new speaker, giving you the maximum amount of flexibility with a minimum of fuss.

When family and friends visit, they sit on the couch and Bill and I pull chairs together. I plunk mine between the sofa and Bill's chair, slightly off center to avoid blocking anyone's line of sight to another's face. In the dining room, I choose a seat in the middle of the dining table, my back to the source of light.

When Bill and I are alone, I lift a lightweight chair from its spot across the living room and place it facing him, the arm of my chair touching his, before we settle down to talk. For brief exchanges, I kneel in front of him, my hands on his knees, or I stand face-to-face about twelve inches from his familiar face.

Long bedtime chats with my head turned to Bill used to give me a crick in my neck. Now I prop myself comfortably on a pile of pillows and face him, lying down with my head next to his waist. I stretch out, with my feet braced up against the wall near his head. We are both comfortable and relaxed.

The furniture in your office can also be arranged to your benefit. You might need two chairs in addition to your desk chair so that you are not forced to talk across a large desk, which often puts as much as six feet between you and your visitor. When your visitor comes in, walk around the desk to greet him or her, and sit in the extra chair. You can easily collect those items that you might need (such as pencils, pens, and note pads) before the meeting and place them on top of your desk, within easy reach. Another alternative is to bring a chair around to the side of your desk, allowing you to be behind your desk and still drastically cut down the distance between you and your visitor.

Also, take a look at the placement of your desk in relation to the door. When you sit at your desk, are you facing the door? If you are not, can you rearrange your office so you are at least partially facing the door? As your hearing loss changes, you may begin to find that a quiet-footed person can enter your office without your knowing it. But what if you cannot move the desk? If the position of your desk is fixed and forces you to keep your back to the entry way, you might consider hanging a small mirror on the wall in front of you, or putting one facing the door on the edge of your desk, in your normal line of sight. This may be unusual, but it really helps.

For those who work in offices that have a conference room, I have only one piece of advice: *use it*. This is especially true for the person who does not have a private office. Conference rooms are often not used on a daily basis, making them the perfect place to talk with several people at once. You can seat yourself in the spot that offers the best lighting and maximum closeness to others. These rooms are usually well lit and are acoustically superior to offices because of their thick carpets, curtains, plush chairs, and often heavy wall coverings or works of art, all of which absorb noise and make communication easier.

Acoustics

Acoustics refers to the way in which specific areas treat sounds. For example, a place with bad acoustics is one in which sounds echo. Bathrooms and kitchens, large workrooms, and many offices send sounds right back at you because of their metal, linoleum, and ceramic surfaces; their bare walls; and their lack of curtains. These areas echo the sounds of the speaker, as well as the sound of a shoe scuffing, a cough, water gurgling, and machines running. These rooms do not contain materials to muffle normal environmental noises, and thus these sounds often interfere with conversation.

Kitchens have the worst acoustics, with basements and bathrooms a very close second. These rooms also have a high level of noise with all those fans, furnaces, refrigerators, and washers and dryers. Doctors' and dentists' treatment rooms, with polished surfaces and bare walls, are also not built for hard of hearing people.

Living rooms, dens, and corporate conference rooms have better acoustics. The cloth and carpet absorb the noises and usually you do not find any machinery running. You can improve the acoustics of these rooms even further. For example, you can cover metal venetian blinds with cloth window shades. If your windows are not curtained, curtain them. Hardwood floors are beautiful, but carpet deadens sounds.

And how about your walls? If you do not have or like framed artwork, one of the most effective things you can do is to find a small rug or a tapestry and use it as a wall hanging. For something unusual, how about copies of American Indian saddle blankets? You can find them at any Western supply store or saddle shop in a variety of designs and colors to suit any style or taste. They absorb the sound that bare walls would shoot right back.

Home Improvements
Dr. Donald Holden

Improving the acoustics of a home to accommodate a hearing-impaired person improves the quality of that person's life. It increases the livability of the home and broadens the hearing-impaired person's opportunities to participate in family activities. Eve points out how much she misses family conversations. When she's not able to understand, she feels like an outsider, distanced from the rest of the family. Being excluded hurts her deeply. Improving the acoustics helps include a hearing-impaired person in the family. That alone can give one a big lift.

Too often in a family, the members feel they have fulfilled their obligations when they acknowledge the problem and sympathize or commiserate. But friends and family members can go beyond that. They can do practical things such as monitor sound quality, make sure that electronic devices are outfitted with lights to increase safety and improve the hearing-impaired member's participation in family life, move furniture to create better conversation areas, or increase lighting. All these actions are inclusionary rather than exclusionary, bringing the hearing-impaired person back into the life of the family, back into the loop of conversation.

At work, if your organization will accommodate your special need, ask for a thick carpet, floor-length drapes, and couple of wall hangings. If you do not have your own office, try landscape partitions covered with thick carpet. If you are not crazy about saddle blankets, you can buy or make painted or silk-screen-print fabric wall hangings that are stretched over frames. They are inexpensive, attractive, and come in all different patterns and styles. They would certainly help.

One misconception you may have heard is that acoustical ceiling tiles make up for a lack of carpet, drapes, fabric-covered chairs, and wall hangings. They do not. They help, but they are not nearly as effective alone as when coupled with fabric that covers as many surfaces as possible.

Are all these changes going to instantly do away with any problem you might have in understanding conversation? No. But they help, regardless of whether you are just beginning to experience problems in communication, or have been dealing with them for years.

In everyday life, too many occasions arise when we are stuck with bad acoustics. My biggest problem was my own reluctance to ask for help. Now I take responsibility for making the first move. I state my needs clearly and move myself to find the best lighting and position near the speaker. This helps overcome those problems caused by bad acoustics. I have more confidence now and am doing much better communicating with those who are important to me.

Background Noise

The hum of appliances, the whir of the air conditioner, the clatter of a nearby typewriter, the blare of traffic, the rattle of dishes, all of these things can affect your ability to understand conversation.

If you want a sense of the background noise in a given place, ask a person with normal hearing to stand quietly and listen for a moment and then to tell you all the different sounds he or she hears. You may be surprised at the answer! If you wear strong hearing aids, you probably can no longer single out one voice from a noisy background, nor can you partially shut out other voices and sounds. You have lost much of the human ear's extraordinary ability to compensate for background noise. In addition, your hearing aids may distort noises, making some unusually loud and others indistinguishable. You need to be aware of this.

Let me describe to you, briefly, how the world sounds and feels to me through my "mechanical ears."

In my kitchen, the dishwasher is as loud as a subway train rushing along underground. At the kitchen sink, water running from the faucets sounds as if I am standing under Niagara Falls and blocks out all other noise. The electric fan over the stove hurts my ears, and I have to turn my hearing aid and my implant speech processor down when I turn the fan on. In our living room, which is acoustically excellent, the sound of the furnace fan in the basement is detectable if I sit near an outlet, and it slightly blurs the speech input I pick up.

Both TVs and stereos interfere with my understanding of speech, although they are not troublesome to my ears. I hear no sounds of music except one note, near Middle C, which is the same tone I hear for all human voices. I do clearly sense the beat of music. I can dance to it and sometimes guess a song from the special pattern of its rhythm. If anyone wants to carry on a conversation with me, we turn off the radio or stereo, because even if they are on low, they interfere. If Bill wants to comment on a TV program or to clue me in on some action or information that I missed, he must turn the sound off for a moment. When the programs are closed-captioned, I am in seventh heaven.

Because you can do nothing about background noise beyond trying to improve the acoustics of your surroundings, you need to become more aware of it and work around it as much as possible. This includes never trying to hold a lengthy conversation in a bathroom or kitchen, a basement, a noisy work area, on a busy street, in a crowded restaurant, or anywhere the combination of background noise and poor acoustics can overwhelm you or interfere with your hearing aid. You must tactfully discourage people from trying to talk to you in such places. Either lead them to a place with better acoustics and less background noise or ask them to wait a moment until the noise subsides. You can explain that the interference is too overwhelming for you, and that you just cannot understand them with such competition.

You may run the risk that others are not willing to understand your communication needs. But if you cannot hear well under poor conditions, if you do not assert your needs, the only person you will hurt is yourself. You will get frustrated and confused, misunderstand parts of the conversation, and perhaps even misrepresent yourself. On the other hand, most people are probably going to be cooperative once they understand the situation.

Dining Out

When Bill and I eat out, we choose restaurants that have the best seating arrangements and acoustics with the least amount of background noise and music. We automatically choose a table near curtains or walls, as far away from busy areas as possible. I sit with my back to the wall and the lighting in my favor.

I read the menu carefully and select my choices before the waiter appears, so I can state my complete order, not waiting for the usual questions concerning choices.

If you are hosting a restaurant meal, you have several choices. First, make sure the waiter understands that you are paying the tab. To keep up with what others are ordering, you might ask one of your guests to relay the others' selections to you. Assistive listening devices, such as directional microphone attachments, can be helpful in these situations, allowing you to pick up as much as you can of the conversation. You can also use pad and pen. The objective is to be comfortable and decisive, to feel that you are in charge, and gracefully so.

When going along with the crowd to a "joint that is jumping," you can still place your orders. Then sit back, relax, eat, and watch. If you are a businessperson who is expected to entertain clients, and someone schedules a meeting at a noisy restaurant, then you may have to get very assertive and take control of not only this situation, but the possibility of similar situations arising in the future.

You may need to take your employer aside and tell him or her that because of background noise, you cannot understand spoken conversation in such settings. "After all," you might say, "you would not expect a person with limited vision to read a computer printout." If the employer wishes you to wine and dine clients, then you must be allowed to choose the restaurant.

Another alternative I've used successfully for business lunches and dinners is to have the meal brought in. Many caterers and some restaurants now prepare and deliver lunches and dinners to business offices. Some of the services even deliver the meal complete with plates, cutlery, and glasses. Yes, it can be expensive to have such deluxe meals delivered, but consider what you might spend at a three- or four-star restaurant and the added benefit of being able to control your environment and to effectively communicate. It may be worth the price.

If you find yourself in this situation often, you might even consider purchasing a complete set of silverware and dishes, napkins, and various types of glasses, even a wine bottle opener, to keep in the office.

Above all, do not be afraid to be different. Experiment, think of new or unusual alternatives to restaurants. Fortunately, Portland is surrounded by beautiful parks. If you are lucky enough to live in a scenic location, why not take an out-of-town visitor on a real picnic, to get out of doors and gaze at a beautiful vista or to rest under a tree by a river or lake? "Eating out" does not necessarily have to mean eating in a restaurant.

Telephone Tactics

Losing the use of the telephone in today's world is devastating. It is worth the effort to learn new tricks and seek out new equipment to ease communication through this vital link.

Telephones and Hearing Aids

Experiment with telephones and your hearing aid. Many people find they do better by turning up the volume of their phone amplifying receiver and removing their hearing aid. Others use the hearing aid with or without the "T-switch" (T for telephone) that is built into many hearing aids. (This is a feature you may want to learn more about before purchasing your first, or next, hearing aid.)

Not all telephones have amplifying receivers, so it pays to know how your hearing aid works best for you. Moving the receiver around your ear and aid as you listen to a telephone conversation will help you find the best possible angle for optimal reception. You will also learn how to avoid the squealing feedback that is caused when the receiver is too close. Try dialing a recorded announcement, such as "time," and playing with all the options available to you. That way you will not be pressured to understand a conversation, and you can just play and experiment until you find what works best for you.

Telephoning in noisy surroundings is sometimes necessary, especially in emergencies. The "T-switch" is then invaluable because it cuts out all background noises. (See the Reference Section for more information on T-switches and amplifiers.)

Making Appointments

Even though our telephone conversations may be restricted to giving out carefully planned information and receiving only limited responses, we can figure out ways to verify the accuracy of these responses.

This is your first lesson in taking control: If you need to make an appointment, take the initiative. Suggest two or three different dates and times that are convenient for you. That way you limit the other person's responses to words you have already spoken ("Tuesday afternoon," "Thursday morning"). When you know in advance what the receptionist might say, you are much more likely to understand her. Here is an example:

> *Eve:* "I'd like an appointment with Mrs. Smith on Wednesday or Thursday afternoon between two and four. Is that possible, please? I'm hard of hearing and will need careful speech."
> *Receptionist:* "How about Thursday at two?"
> *Eve:* "Did you say 'Thursday'?"
> *Receptionist:* "Yes, I did."
> *Eve:* "And did you say 'three'?"
> *Receptionist:* "No, I said 'Two.'"
> *Eve:* "I'll be there at two o'clock Thursday. Is that correct? Good. Thank you so much for your patience."

Personal Calls

Personal calls, especially sensitive ones, are trickier. We want to convey our messages graciously and then offer others comfortable responses. As an example, if I am phoning a friend who is grieving over the loss of a family member, I might ask, "Would you like me to come over? I'll be able to understand you if you answer either, 'That would be nice,' or 'Thank you, but I'm busy right now.'" These two choices differ enough in sound and length to make it easy for me to understand the response and are gracious enough so neither of us feels embarrassed, as we would be if we used abrupt answers such as *yes* or *no.*

One-word, one-syllable responses, such as *yeah, no, right, wrong,* and *here,* are the hardest to understand when you cannot see the speaker's mouth. Yet it is natural for others to use the shortest possible response because they think long-winded answers will be overwhelming, and they are quite right. It is best to shoot for medium-length answers—"Yes, that would be nice," "Yes, I'd like that very much," "No, that's not possible right now. (Pause.) How about tomorrow?"

The most difficult part of taking an incoming call is figuring out who's calling. If you are losing the ability to identify voices over the phone, even your nearest and dearest may give you too few clues. "Hi, this is Bob" may not be enough information for you to recognize your own brother.

One way to set an example, and then ask others to do the same for you, is to answer the phone with your own full name. The caller's full name in return will usually provide enough syllables for you to identify the person.

When my phone rings, I say, "Hi. This is Eve Nickerson." If the caller then repeats back to me either my first or last name, I will have an important clue as to whether or not this person knows me well and a little extra time to adjust to the caller's voice. My family and friends know how well this works, which encourages me to suggest it to each new person who has reason to telephone me. One of my friends always responds, "Eve, this is Elizabeth Hirsch." My younger daughter responds, "Mommy, this is your daughter Kay." Our accountant says, "Mrs. Nickerson, this is Alice Gannet, your accountant from Jensen and Jensen."

If a caller greets my opening with, "This is Herb," and I have no idea what name was said, I will ask for his full name. Even then, I am often lost. If this happens, then I ask, "Can you give me your full name again, please? If I can't figure out who you are, I'll turn on my answering service, and you can call me back and state your name and message. Then I'll call you back, if necessary."

Sales pitches, whether live or prerecorded, are easy to identify. If a voice starts a quick spiel, I interrupt after three sentences. "Excuse me, but I'm hard of hearing. If this call is important, please call me back in five minutes. I'll put my phone on to the answering service." Anyone really needing to reach me does so. A prerecorded message will keep right on talking away through my interruption. If that happens, I hang up.

All Alone with No Help in Sight

All this good advice is not to imply that I have never been caught with no help at all. One time when Bill doubled over with pain, and I drove that familiar route to the hospital emergency room, I forgot to put the slip-on telephone amplifier into my purse.

Six hours later, after the surgeons had wheeled him into the operating theater, I looked around me for help in telephoning our children and neighbors. The corridors were empty. Worrying, I stuck my quarter into the pay phone, and put the receiver to my ear with the cochlear implant—the only device I had that would pick up a dial tone and some semblance of human voices without an amplifier. No sound. The rechargeable battery had run down. In my haste, I had not put a charged one in my purse.

I hung up, and my quarter came back. I took a deep breath and struggled for control. I put the quarter back in, counted to five, hoping that was long enough for the dial tone. Then I dialed our daughter Twink's number from my emergency sheet (all numbers having departed my spinning brain). Again I counted to five, trusting that by then she had answered and had begun to talk.

"Twink, this is Mom. I'm on a public phone and can't hear you. Don't worry." I repeated that three times, to give her time to answer the phone. Then I described the circumstances, told her I was going to repeat the whole message, did so, told her, "I love you," and hung up.

I repeated this process with Kay, asking her to phone Allen and Elaine long distance as well. By now I was feeling more confident. I phoned my neighbor so she would not worry as the day darkened into night.

Each of them later thanked me for the message. It had worked just fine with no friendly stranger nor effective audio equipment to help.

Emergencies

Staying calm in emergencies is doubly difficult if telephoning is a problem. What little we may understand over the phone in the best of circumstances is jeopardized by stress. To help me, a police dispatch officer and an emergency room doctor put their heads together and wrote the following script for me:

(Dial 911, or your local emergency numbers. Keep the list with the script.)
This is Eve Nickerson.
I am hard of hearing. I will repeat this whole message at the end.
(State the Problem)
Our house is on fire, (or)
My husband is dangerously ill, (or)
An auto accident on our street, (etc.).
(State Your Needs, if necessary.)
Fire engine, (or)

Ambulance, life support systems, CPR, etc., (or)
Police, (etc.).
Our address is _____.
(Write it out. Don't trust your memory.)
Our telephone number is _____. (Again, write it out.)
Our nearest cross-street or intersection is. (State it.)
Our porch light will be on. (In medical emergencies.)
The front door will be unlocked.
We will be on the second floor. (Or wherever.)
Now I will repeat everything I said, because I can't hear you.
(Repeat from top.)

Both the police dispatch officer and the emergency room doctor warned us to repeat the message in its entirety. Often, they said, an emergency dispatcher may miss an important piece of information. Since we will not understand their questions, repeating the entire message is the safest means to success. They both emphasized that in most cases, an extra thirty seconds will have little effect on the danger we are facing, and it may make all the difference in getting effective help.

I have printed this information in large, black letters (easy to read without glasses) on pieces of cardboard and put them by all three of our phones. On the back, I printed telephone numbers of our doctors, our family members, and our neighbors.

Safe Driving

Many adults who lose their hearing worry that they also will lose their driver's license; however, a license to drive noncommercial vehicles cannot reasonably be withheld from a hearing-impaired person. Now that I am over sixty-five, I must apply in person for my license renewal in the state of Oregon. Each time, I point to the back of the renewal form, where one must make a check mark for any known handicap. I explain how much I can hear of important sounds (horns, sirens, etc.) and how I use my eyes, and then I brace myself, prepared to defend my rights by argument or by hiring an attorney.

Each time, I have gone away laughing at my keyed-up emotions. I have met with no problems and no handicapped check marks, only pleasant smiles and my renewed license.

However, my own concern for safe driving is constant. I remind myself to watch all my rear view mirrors, to pay strict attention to the scene around me, and to be a polite and defensive driver.

If I have passengers, I explain ahead of time that I can talk to them, but they should not try to respond with long sentences. Since I understand little without seeing their faces, this is strictly a one-sided operation. On long drives, we take turns not only driving, but talking; I watch their mouths instead of the scenery. We work out hand signals ahead of time in case they have urgent messages to tell me (a necessary stop, or new directions). I can then pull over at a safe stopping place to communicate. With more than one passenger, I smilingly tell them to talk to each other and not to worry about me. It all works just fine.

Travel Tips

Hearing-impaired people who travel frequently have their own tricks to smooth the way, pleasantly alerting airport personnel and flight attendants, bus drivers, station masters, or fellow travelers ahead of time to their needs or concerns. On well-known routes, routines are so well-established that little need be said. Even so, the most experienced traveler can still end up in Portland, Maine, instead of Portland, Oregon. To avoid unexpected cross-country trips, I always take the following steps.

First, when making reservations, I inform people that I am hard of hearing. This information is entered into the computer. I will be contacted or found if there is a change of plans, since loudspeaker announcements are meaningless static to me.

Second, I tell personnel at boarding areas that I am hard of hearing and sit within sight of them. If important announcements are made over the loud speaker, I need someone to come and tell me. I also ask people next to me to keep me informed of changes or boarding arrangements.

Third, when boarding, I always ask the attendant, "Is this the plane or train or bus going to Portland, *Oregon?*"

When I am alone on unfamiliar routes, I keep one, five, and ten dollar bills folded in half and tucked in a ready pocket, handy for porters and attendants who have steered me through unfamiliar stations and airports. Fellow travelers have been wonderfully helpful, cheerfully interpreting loud speaker announcements concerning boardings, delays, and ever-dreaded cancellations.

Guided tours are not normally planned for hearing-impaired travelers, and we tend to avoid them because we cannot understand the guides and the lectures. To help us, Self Help for the Hard of Hearing, Inc., has begun providing packaged tours especially for us (see Reference Section).

Living Alone

For those who are living alone, every problem or solution we talk about in this book may be a higher obstacle to hurdle, a shakier bridge to cross, or a deeper pit out of which to crawl.

For many years, we have learned from our hearing-impaired friends how valiantly they have battled alone; how discouraged they have become; how many times they have picked themselves up, brushed off their frustrations and fears, and set out once more to work their way back into the hearing world, which is inhabited by almost everyone they know.

Although we have written this book from the enviable surroundings of a loving family, some day each of us may be alone. We hope for the courage to reach out instead of to withdraw, the strength to push ourselves to find solutions to our problems, and the self-discipline to keep struggling until we make those solutions work.

We know there is no standing still to rest on our laurels. We either move forward or go backward. We pray that all of us, despite that one backward step we always seem to take, can still keep taking those two steps forward.

Four

Communication Beyond Words

Although communication includes hearing the words, Kay has taught me that there is *much* more to it than that: The way we listen can have a profound impact on our ability to understand.

Stay Calm

If there is any one key to understanding speech better, that key would be to *relax*. Getting upset will get you nowhere—fast. Communication is a complex interaction, something that we tend to take for granted until a hearing loss makes us realize just how difficult it is. In order to understand as much as possible under adverse conditions, we need to bring intelligence to bear on the problem.

When I am relaxed and happy, my ability to understand is at its highest. If I am tired, depressed, upset, or anxious, my ability to understand is impaired: If I am a little upset, I will miss a few key words; if I am very upset, I will miss a lot of words; if I am tired, depressed, and upset, I will miss almost all of them. Here is a simple guide to follow: If you have a 50 percent hearing loss in the frequencies of normal speech, you are approximately 50 percent less likely to understand speech, given the best of conditions. If you are tired, add 10 percent, and if you are feeling "down," add another 10 percent. If you are straining to catch every word rather than the message, add another 10 percent. And if all this makes you feel upset, strained, and irritable, add another 10 percent. If you are experiencing all of these things, in a perfectly controlled environment, such as a soundproof room, listening to a person who enunciates clearly, you may only be likely to understand 10 percent.

Now I am certainly not saying you should always run around with a smile pinned to your face. We all have days that are better than others. We need to be aware that our emotions can greatly contribute to or impair our ability to understand. Therefore, we must adjust our expectations, activities, or both, accordingly. Also, by being aware of the problem, we can begin to control it.

If I don't understand the speaker, I step back and take a deep breath. Then, I let the speaker know that he has lost me, and I ask him to please back up and start again. If I still don't get it, I try to laugh. I might say something like, "Well, I'm *still* not getting it. Can you tell me what the topic is?" Usually, with the topic made clear, I catch on better. And because I did not allow the situation to upset me, I will be able to continue to get the maximum amount of information available.

Do Not Try to Understand Every Word

This may seem rather strange at first, but when I try to hear every single word, I end up hearing or understanding *less* than if I just relax and understand the words that I do hear.

All languages include many words that do not carry much meaning. Sometimes these words just provide a structure for other words—for example, the word *of* in the prepositional phrase "of my best friends." Other times they are count nouns, words we use to count other words, such as *group* of friends, *grains* of sand, or *flock* of birds. Or, they are words that we do not really need to understand a message correctly, such as *a, the, and,* and sometimes, verbs such as *is.*

I try to remember that I do not need to hear every single word to understand the message. Much of the time, the rhythm of the sentence will tell me that I did not hear a couple of words, but I can still guess the meaning of the whole sentence because I can use my knowledge of how language works and the topic being discussed to fill in the words that are missing. Often those missing words (the short, one syllable words) are the hardest to hear anyway.

So the upshot of the matter is that, instead of concentrating on each and every word, I concentrate on the message, using all the information available to me to understand that message. This includes being aware of my surroundings and of the person who is talking. There are times, of course, when we must understand all the important words, especially when conducting personal and professional business. But for most day-to-day social conversation, we only need to get close (and, in some cases, sort-of-close may be good enough).

Most of the time, communicating with someone, exchanging information, is not so much a matter of getting all the words right. Goodness knows, nobody is perfect at choosing just the right word every time. Communication consists of moving a message from person to person. Sometimes I need only a few of the words to understand the message, and sometimes I need none at all. But I almost never need every single one. It is the message that counts, not the words.

While this is very easy for us to say, believe me, I understand how hard it is to do. As I lost my ability to hear, I tried harder and harder to catch every single word in order to understand. I focused more and more of my energy and my intellect on getting all the words correctly. But the harder I concentrated on the words, the less I understood the speaker's message because I was wasting energy on the words *all, the, in,* and *this* rather than *flowers, smell, garden,* and *year.* These words are just enough to let me know what the speaker is talking about, which is, "All the flowers in the garden smell so nice this year."

Ask for the Topic

If you find yourself totally lost whether from someone's quick directions or an involved conversation, one of the easiest ways to get back on track is to ask, What are we talking about? or What's the topic? (This is so important that we will go into it in detail in chapter 7.)

For the moment, imagine this scene. You and two friends are enjoying a conversation about your respective vacation plans. Suddenly, your friends begin an animated discussion. You are immediately confused. After four sentences are exchanged, the only words you have picked up are, "Did you hear . . .?" and "How exciting!"

As soon as they stop to catch their breath, you smile and ask in an amused voice, "What *are* you talking about?"

"Oh, I'm sorry. Jean asked me if I'd heard that Ellen is going to have a baby."

"Oh, how wonderful! Tell us more," you reply.

Automatically their faces turn toward you, and now with the topic clear, you understand the words. In addition, you have preserved the pleasant atmosphere (and your friendships) by keeping your voice clear of any reproach while asking for more information to fill in what you missed, rather than troubling them for an exact repetition.

The problems begin with the fact that I simply do not hear all the words being spoken, so I am easily confused when I hear words that do not make any sense.

Everyone loses the topic of conversation at some point. Our minds wander, we do not pay attention as well as we should. For people like myself, though, losing the topic is a disaster. We are only getting one in three or five or ten words anyway. But if we know the topic, we can manage to follow along in a great many situations. Therefore, it is vital that we ask for the topic the minute we realize that we have lost it.

In our family we have developed a hand signal that I can use. When several of us are talking and I lose the thread of the conversation, I make a *T* with my hands (the same signal football and basketball players use to ask for a time-out during a game). The person nearest to me will clue me in on the current topic, and off we go. The trick is to have some sort of system that works for you and those around you. That way you can relax, knowing that if you need it, help is near at hand.

Use Paper and Pen

Pulling out a pad and pen, or keeping them handy on a desk or table, is an obvious device. It is indispensable when making dates, appointments, or notes of important facts to remember. When another person is giving me such information, it is much wiser for that person to write it down for me, or see to it that I do so.

When Bill tells me that the Johnsons and the Smiths are coming to dinner next week, and I have nothing handy to write with, he has learned to distrust my response if I say, "That's nice." I probably heard something quite different such as, "John and Midge are going on a trip next week." If the information is important, he now asks me to repeat back exactly what he said. If I get it wrong, he says it again. We sometimes go into a repeat-and-repeat-back dialogue that sounds like the famous Abbot and Costello routine "Who's on first?" This is awkward and annoying, but it is far less embarrassing than having four hungry people arrive unexpectedly on our doorstep.

The greater my hearing loss, the more I forget even the most important information if it is not repeated or written down. This has done nothing to improve my morale. After Kay explained the reason for my forgetfulness (see chapter 9), I could set aside my bruised feelings and go about finding corrective measures, the best of which has proven to be a half dozen small spiral notebooks with pens attached by rubber bands, scattered about the house and in my purses.

I have no reservations about pulling out written material at business conferences and certainly not in hospitals. Five times in five years, I rushed Bill to the emergency rooms of Portland hospitals. I learned to carry with me diagrams of his previous surgeries, lists of his medications, and a quick summary of his immediate symptoms. Then, I watched and waited. It was easy enough to tell when doctors and nurses, after busily attaching tubes, were still looking for answers by taking tests, comparing old and new X-rays and ultrasound pictures. When the consulting was done and the decisions made, I approached the doctor who seemed to be in charge and asked, "What's wrong, and what are you going to do?"

"Oh, I forgot you couldn't hear us!"

"I don't expect you to remember. Bill needed your attention, not me. Just draw me a picture." And they always did, with careful explanations.

In spite of these experiences, it took me a long time to pull out my pad and pen at a luncheon or dinner table. Even though my friends were often perceptive and loving enough to use their own paper and pen for me, I felt it was both an imposition on them and an embarrassment to me.

Today, my pad and pen sit on snowy white table cloths at formal dinners and banquets. They get passed back and forth at luncheons and are always at hand in my purse or pocket for emergencies. In one month, when I thanked six people at three separate functions for using their notes and making it easier for me, each one said, "But it's so much easier for us, too!"

Spell Out Loud

There are times when paper and pen are not at hand. If I miss a person's name or the name of a place that someone is describing to me, which I usually do, I ask the speaker to spell it out loud. "Spell it, please," is quickly said.

At first, I had difficulty remembering the letters of words longer than four letters, unless they were common words or names such as *Smith*. I was discouraged, yet people's names are so important to both them and me that I began to practice in front of a mirror. I spoke the letters of the alphabet, noticing how they looked on my mouth. That helped. The next time I asked that a name be spelled, I quickly repeated each letter back. That helped too. Soon my mind seemed to stretch its ability to retain the letters, to group them, to make sense of them. It was well worth the effort.

If you want to learn the basics of lipreading, contact your local community college or hospital hearing clinic, or ask your hearing aid dealer or audiologist (if you have one) where to find tutors or classes in your vicinity. If you prefer self-study and own a VCR, I recommend a series of videotapes entitled "Read My Lips" (see the Reference Section for more details).

Hearing Aids

Hearing aids or other electronic devices are critical to my ability to communicate. But they have limitations. Sometimes the limitations reside in the equipment. Hearing aids are wonderful, but they are far from perfect. Some of the biggest limitations, however, are inside ourselves.

We all have to jump three hurdles in order to use modern electronic devices, such as hearing aids: First, we are reluctant to admit to a hearing loss since it signals a problem we would rather not face. Second, we are reluctant to purchase hearing aids (we have heard too many others complain about them). And third, we are reluctant to wear hearing aids because they are embarrassing and annoying and because their tiny dials and batteries can be hard to handle.

Nevertheless, many electronic devices are available to assist hard of hearing people. While not perfect, these devices are really wonderful when used effectively. Many hearing aids now come with a basic instruction booklet that will help you understand and operate them. But the booklets do not tell you everything.

Beyond the Instruction Booklet

One of the most important pieces of advice I can give you is to see a doctor first, preferably an ear, nose, and throat specialist or an otologist (ear specialist). If you have not seen one, think about going now. A hearing loss can derive from a variety of causes—ranging from something as simple as impacted wax blocking the ear canal to complex problems, such as deterioration in the tiny bones in the middle ear, or to damage to the nerves of the inner ear. It pays to know what you are dealing with and whether the problem can be corrected by a medical procedure or treatment, either now or perhaps in the future.

Once you and your hearing aid dealer have decided on the aid most likely to help you, ask to use the aid for a trial period of at least two weeks before final purchase. Keep a diary or records that describe your experiences and sensations that you will then discuss with your dealer. You may need an adjustment or even a different type of hearing aid altogether. Hearing aids are expensive, and you have a right to find out if you are getting the very best one for your particular hearing loss. Remember too that it may take time to adapt to the increase in all the sound and noise that you receive through your aid.

This seems to be a Catch 22. If this is your first hearing aid, how will you know if it is the best one for you when you have not yet adapted to the sound you hear through your hearing aid? This is where good record-keeping and a reputable, hardworking hearing aid dealer play a key role. If the hearing aid dealer understands as precisely as possible what problems you are having under what conditions, the dealer can determine, based on his or her experience and expertise, whether or not you are getting optimal performance from the aid. But you must contribute good records of your problems and successes, and you need to choose a hearing aid dealer with all the care and attention that you use to choose your doctor.

If your hearing aid earmold is not a perfect fit, it can cause soreness or create squealing "feedback" noise in the microphone. A reputable hearing aid dealer can correct this problem and, in my experience, without charge.

Once you have a hearing aid and have worn it for a while, you may find that the volume needs to be manually adjusted for maximum comfort. For the most part, you need to remember that the people who manufacture and fit or implant these hearing devices do not wear them themselves. Also, no two people are the same, so take recommended settings with a grain of salt. Use common sense and find the setting that gives you the most sound possible and yet is still comfortable. This setting can change depending on the amount and loudness of background noise, what you are trying to hear, or with whom you are trying to communicate. It can even depend on how you feel. The more tired you are, the less tolerant you may be to noise, so turn the volume down a bit if it bothers you. If you need to hear something, you can always turn it back up.

Hearing and Hearing Aids

Dr. Donald Holden

A whole range of electronic devices is available today to help hard of hearing people. Adjustments can also be made to equipment or devices in the home to make them accessible. For example, the telephone can be adjusted so that the ring is louder, the pattern of the ring can be altered to attract attention, or a flashing light signal can be attached to the phone so that the hard of hearing person can know when the phone is ringing. Intercoms have varying combinations and degrees of special features as do electronic surveillance systems. All of these offer convenience and protection and are available with a wide range of features and price. These devices enhance the efficiency of communication to make daily living more pleasant and less harried.

We are all familiar with hearing aids for they are becoming more and more commonplace. It should be sta⁺ed at the outset that not everyone can use a hearing aid effectively or with pleasure. The reasons are many and have to do with human nature on the one hand and the limitations of hearing aids on the other hand.

We human beings are a marvelous mixture of pride, sensitivity, and prejudice, among other things. No one likes to advertise a handicap and wearing a hearing aid is an admission that the wearer has a hearing problem. This can be a blow to one's pride. The same psychological rejection is at work here as it is in the refusal of some people with vision problems to wear glasses. The antidote is to accept the fact that no human is totally perfect—we must accept ourselves as we are if we hope to have a healthy psyche. Then, we must find the ways and means to help ourselves overcome our deficiencies. Using a hearing aid to improve one's hearing, when that is possible, can open the door to happier and easier living, for without communication, we are all made poorer.

Another deterrent for some people is the cost of hearing aids. We all know people who have hearing aids and then do not use them or use them only on occasion, all the while complaining that the hearing aids are not suitable for one reason or another. To a person with limited financial means, this is a powerful argument against purchasing a hearing aid. Frankly, all too often a poor match is made between the hearing aid and the presumed wearer. Some hearing aid dealers will sell hearing aids to anyone and everyone who will pay the price, whether the instrument is appropriate or not. Naturally, this causes great bitterness and disappointment. Fortunately, efforts are under way to regulate the industry so that these abuses are minimized. And the situation is improving.

People who need a hearing aid but cannot afford it should not give up on the idea, though. Many teaching institutions and large clinics collect used hearing aids, and they can adapt these aids at little or no cost to a new owner. Medical societies and social service agencies usually know of these possibilities and can direct someone to them.

Finally, a number of people resist the use of hearing aids because they find hearing aids to be annoying, somewhat difficult to handle, sometimes uncomfortable to wear, and often quirky to insert. Changing the battery in a hearing aid can be a daunting exercise to a person with severe arthritis or loss of manual dexterity. Some hearing-impaired people develop a fixation with their hearing aids and constantly play with them, causing the ears to become sensitive, tender, or even inflamed and infected. In these situations, a visit to the trusted audiologist, hearing aid dealer, or ear specialist will resolve the problem. And it is a good idea to have another member of the family or a friend take over inserting the hearing aids when the task seems beyond reach.

Today, most hearing aids come with an instruction booklet that covers the basic "what to do" and "what not to do" with the hearing aid to get the best results. However, several considerations need to be addressed.

In the first place, anyone with a hearing problem should consult an otolaryngologist (ear, nose, and throat specialist) or otologist (ear, nose, and throat subspecialist) to have a thorough examination of the ear, including a hearing test and whatever else is needed (for example, an X-ray examination or selected laboratory work) in order to precisely define the nature of the hearing loss. These physician specialists have an M.D. degree plus postgraduate training to prepare them as experts in problems of the ears and hearing. Do not settle for less. Furthermore, these specialists are not equally expert in all areas. Consult your local medical society and hospital, and if there is a local medical teaching facility, consult the department of otolaryngology there. In this way you can become aware of the background preparation and experience of the specialist you seek.

When you are searching for a specialist, it is a good idea to have several possible candidates in mind. That way you don't have to start the search all over again if your first choice turns out to be less desirable than you supposed. Try to find a specialist you feel you can trust and in whom you can have confidence, someone who will listen to your troubles and care about you. You will have a long professional association with this person and not regret the time you took to select the proper physician.

A second consideration you must make is whether to consult an audiologist or a hearing aid dealer if you need a hearing aid. Your ear specialist can give you good advice in your selection.

If you decide to go to an audiologist for your hearing tests, once again check with your specialist and the Society of Audiologists to be sure you are in good hands. In addition to testing your hearing, the audiologist can recommend hearing aids and then provide assistance to help you adjust to wearing the aids. Ask to see the audiologist's certification from the American Speech-Language-Hearing Association. Certified audiologists have completed a master's degree in audiology, passed a national examination, and have completed supervised training.

It is important that you know as much as possible about the nature and consequences of your hearing problem and the options that are open to you. Top-grade professionals can steer you in the right direction and help you avoid pitfalls that could cause greater difficulties. Whether the treatment you need is clinical, medical, or surgical, and whether you should consider a hearing aid or some other device, you can have confidence and trust in your carefully selected professionals. This goes a long way to allay your anxiety and fears.

Generally, hearing aids come as two types: air conduction and bone conduction. Air conduction aids are by far the more common. They can be fitted entirely in the ear, or behind the ear. If these hearing aids are properly selected and fitted, they are helpful. Prices will vary with the power and quality of the aid, but as a rule, comparable aids from different manufacturers will be comparable in price and performance.

All air conduction hearing aids amplify sound and use the natural mechanisms of the ear to move that sound from the outer to the inner ear to the auditory nerve (the nerve of hearing). This means that the sound has to pass through the middle ear from the eardrum (tympanic membrane) to the oval window by way of the three ossicles (bones) that form a chain—the malleus (hammer), the incus (anvil), and the stapes (stirrup). The stapes fits precisely into and hides the oval window. The vibrations in the middle ear cause the fluid in the inner ear to vibrate, which stimulates the nerve cells in the inner ear and creates electrical impulses that are transmitted to the brain. In the process, the energy of the sound changes from mechanical motion to fluid motion to nerve stimulus.

Ultimately, the auditory nerve determines the level of hearing function. If the nerve is dead, there will be no hearing regardless of the condition of the other parts of the ear. No hearing aid can do anything to overcome the failure of a dead nerve. This is why it is so difficult to help people with nerve deafness. The potential for hearing is limited to the performance of the auditory nerve, and the more damaged the nerve is, the less the hearing can be improved, regardless of the hearing aid, medical therapy, or surgery. The buyer of a hearing aid must beware of promises to correct nerve (sensorineural) deafness and refuse to do business with a seller who advertises such nonsense.

Too often people who purchase hearing aids become frustrated and disappointed because hearing aid dealers have built up their expectations far more than reality can support. When hearing aid purchasers do not get the help they expected from the aids, they feel betrayed and exploited, and rightly so. Let it be stated that the best people in the hearing aid industry—fortunately the majority—are just as appalled as the buyer who is "taken," and they are trying hard to improve the standards and ethics of the industry. Meanwhile, let the buyer beware.

Some hearing losses are a combination of some degree of sensorineural deafness and conductive hearing loss (impaired function of the eardrum and the ossicles). In these complex cases, the advice and expertise of the professionals are most important in providing help and opening a way to improved hearing, better communication, and a happier life. Each person must be evaluated on an individual basis, included in the decision-making process, and approached with total honesty and compassion.

Bone conduction hearing aids are rarely used. These hearing aids by-pass the normal transmission of sound through the middle ear by placement of the aid on the temporal bone behind the external ear so that the sound is transmitted through the bone directly to the auditory nerve. Obviously, these aids are most helpful in those instances that preclude using the normal chain of sound transmission through the middle ear. However, it is difficult to keep bone conduction aids properly placed on the temporal bone, and efforts to do so require some sort of band over the head that is uncomfortable and an almost constant bother.

Luckily, other options are available today. Cross-over arrangements provide a microphone that picks up sound on the side of the poor ear and transmits the sound across to the better ear. This is particularly useful when there is a marked disparity in the two ears. The most recent development is implanted aids that are placed under the skin of the temporal scalp in the best position to receive sound and transmit that sound through the bone to the auditory nerve. And for those people with profound hearing loss in both ears, an implanted multiple channel electrode can be placed part way into the cochlear channel of the ear (cochlear implant). The cochlear implant also has a receiver that is implanted under the skin and an assortment of processors to program the sound.

This does not mean that a solution to deafness is at hand. Far from it. But it does mean that a search is on for improved hearing for those who need it and new advances offer hope and help where none existed before. So do not despair. Seek the best professional help available, establish a good rapport with those in whom you entrust your care, and carefully consider the options open to you. Finally, do not let your expectations outrun reality because to go down that road is to engage in a hopeless search for a miracle. The anguish and pain of such a journey should be avoided.

Also remember that hearing aids are not perfect instruments and that researchers are constantly exploring ways to improve them (just think of the strides that have been made since the old hearing trumpets were introduced). But even the present marvels of electronic circuitry have their shortcomings. For one thing, hearing aids pick up most of the sound available to them and not just the sounds you want to hear. They function best when background noise is absent or minimal and when you can focus, one on one, with another person. If the background noise is impossible to tolerate or too confusing, or if there is a chance that a sudden noise (such as a blast on a horn, a dropped tray of glasses, or an explosion) can occur, please turn off your hearing aid. And if you are dining out or are otherwise troubled by extraneous sound, it is a good idea to rely on speechreading so that communication can proceed without interference. Many books, videotapes, and classes are available to help you develop your speechreading skills.

The proper fitting of hearing aids is important both for comfort and efficiency. Be sure that you are satisfied with the fit and work with your hearing aid dealer or audiologist until things are right. Once you have properly fitting hearing aids and have adjusted to them, you will need to keep the aids in good working order. Here are a few suggestions:

- Make sure your hearing aids are completely turned off when you think they are.
- Remove the hearing aids when you go to bed, and remove the batteries when you are not wearing the aids.
- Always carry extra batteries with you.
- Keep a supply of batteries in your freezer or refrigerator.
- Do not get your hearing aids wet.
- Clean your earmolds regularly to remove ear wax.
- Consult your audiologist, hearing aid dealer, or ear specialist when a problem develops, for it is easier and simpler to deal with problems early on rather than later.

Hearing aids are rather complicated instruments and their usefulness depends upon proper care and maintenance along with an attitude adjustment if the best results are to be achieved. You cannot just put them on and forget about them. When rightly understood and used and properly cared for, hearing aids can pay rich dividends. Expert advice and help are at hand to assist hearing aid wearers toward that goal. Do not let yourself be persuaded one way or another by a friend, family member, neighbor, or stranger, no matter how well meaning they might be. The problem is your problem and it is different from that of another person. So, for your own sake, take heed of the suggestions included here to deal with it and you will not be sorry.

You must also keep in mind that each person's hearing loss is unique. You or your family may wonder, as I did, why you cannot do as well as another person with a similar level of hearing loss. I finally learned that my friends and I have hearing losses in different ranges, and in some cases, these losses are of a different kind. Some people lose the higher frequencies; others lose the same number of frequencies, but in a different range. While both types of hearing loss may result in the same percentage of loss on a test, one person may handle voice communication fairly well, while another may have lots of difficulties communicating.

Some kinds of hearing loss are more easily helped than others or respond better to the electronic aids available today. Two people wearing the same kind of hearing aid will not receive the same benefits.

For many, hearing aids distort sound and make it different from our recollection of normal hearing. It is important to talk these concerns over with your audiologist, your ear, nose, and throat physician (ENT), or your hearing aid dealer. Ask for a copy of each one of your audiograms (that is, a chart of your hearing loss). Keep these safe for future reference. Ask each professional to explain your hearing loss and what it means to your understanding of speech and of your environment. Will you miss high frequency sounds, like the *s* and *t* of speech, high notes like the flute or bird songs, or the whine of motors? Or will you miss lower frequencies, such as men's deep voices? Each professional will have different information to share with you, so learn as much as you can. Remember, each of us is different, and what is wonderful for me might be horrid for you. We need to ask questions: How much distortion is unavoidable? How much or what can be done to minimize it?

Hearing Aids and Expectations

Wearing a hearing aid is too often equated with wearing glasses. This is not a happy or correct analogy; it causes too many misconceptions and raises expectations too high. Consider this: A person who has a vision problem can obtain eyeglasses or contact lenses that will correct vision to 20/20 again. By wearing eyeglasses, the person will be able to see as well as most other people.

Wearing a hearing aid does not produce the same results. First of all, hearing aids do not correct most hearing losses. If a person suffers from nerve damage, a hearing aid will not and cannot magically regenerate, repair, or restore the nerves. A hearing aid cannot repair a damaged ear drum, eliminate tinnitus, or reconstruct a cochlea.

Imagine the ear, the entire structure including the middle and inner ear, as if it were a phonograph record. Now, let's damage that record. We will suppose that certain higher sounds are no longer possible and will remove all the sounds on that record above a certain point, say C above middle C. Now, let's try to play that record. As you can see, no matter how sophisticated our stereo system, no matter how high we turn up the volume, we will not hear those high notes because the record, itself, has been damaged. This simulates the problem of profound, selective nerve damage.

Another problem could be that those nerves hear sounds, but they are damaged, so they do not hear those sounds well. Our record will play the higher sounds, but they will be faint in comparison with all of the rest of the sounds on our record. To hear those higher sounds, you would have to turn up the stereo volume fairly high. When you turn up the volume to hear those higher sounds, all the other sounds are also equally as loud. This problem is particularly widespread for the hearing aid wearer. As you can imagine, the more you crank up the volume, the greater the distortion of the sounds that are audible since they are now abnormally amplified.

Hearing aids are limited. They cannot amplify only certain sounds, cannot distinguish between conversation and environmental noise, and without manual adjustment, cannot amplify only some of the time. If a noise occurs within its programmed range, that noise will be amplified, whether it be a dishwasher, a car backfiring, or two cats fighting.

Now you can see why wearing a hearing aid can be so very bothersome, confusing, irritating, or for some people, just plain horrible. Then why, some might ask, should a person even consider purchasing an aid and trying to learn to wear it? Good question. Here is my answer: A hearing loss may not, probably will not, be stable. Here again, we can get into deep trouble if we try to equate a hearing problem with a vision problem. Vision problems often are stable to a certain extent. For example, Kay became nearsighted in the seventh grade. While she has become more nearsighted over time, she will always be nearsighted. She may develop astigmatism, but she will not suddenly become farsighted. Her vision will change, but very slowly, bit by bit.

Having a hearing loss can be, to my mind, much more like having arthritis, in that the severity of the problem can change fairly quickly. Arthritis can be worse on some days more than on other days, at the beginning of the day, after working hard, or on a rainy day. It may be pretty much the same for years, then all of a sudden, it might get much worse. A hearing loss is, in a way, like that for several reasons.

Fatigue plays a very important role in a person's ability to understand spoken communication (see Section II). A person who is tired cannot decode speech as well as one who is fresh. The mind does not process the information as efficiently, which creates the illusion that one did not hear what was said.

Head congestion from a cold or allergy can also diminish one's ability to hear well. While a person with normal hearing usually has little difficulty hearing through a cold, I have a rough time of it. The added problem of a cold or allergy could be just enough to push one over the edge, making it almost impossible to understand much except under perfectly controlled conditions.

And lastly, a hearing loss can be compounded. A person may first experience a hearing loss because of a problem with the mechanisms that conduct sound to the inner ear (especially the bones of the middle ear). Then, one or two or ten years later, the person may suffer the loss of nerve sensitivity in the inner ear. Or that person may also notice a "ringing" in the ears, signaling the onset of tinnitus. Another person, who has experienced the onset of some nerve damage, may find, as time goes on, that more and more hearing is deteriorating. This person never knows, from week to week, month to month, just how much she will be able to hear.

There are those lucky few whose hearing loss is fairly stable, which enables them to wear the same hearing aid with good results for a number of years. This is not, however, something that most people with a hearing loss can necessarily count on.

Many people put off getting a hearing aid when they first realize they have a hearing loss. This is unfortunate because it is much easier to adjust to a hearing aid when the loss is first discovered. Once the hearing loss increases or is compounded with other problems, learning to use a hearing aid effectively could take years. Yes, years.

If you are one of those people who put it off, then go immediately to your doctor or audiologist to have your ears rechecked. If your doctor tells you that your problem is not correctable by a medical procedure, make an appointment with an audiologist or a reputable hearing aid dealer and get a hearing aid. Then start wearing it, start getting used to it. Learn how and when to use it. If you are experiencing tinnitus, contact the American Tinnitus Association and find a doctor or clinic that will help you explore what can be done for you (for additional information, see the Reference Section).

Whatever your hearing problem, one thing is certain—for best results in dealing with your problem you need to get help *now*. Time is not on your side.

Choosing a Hearing Aid Dealer

A hearing aid dealer should be chosen with as much care as a primary care physician. In all probability, the relationship with your hearing aid dealer will be a long one. Make sure it's a good one, too.

You will notice that I did not say, "Choose your hearing aid with care." While this is very important, of key importance is your hearing aid dealer. You want to choose someone who carries many different makes or models of hearing aids since you want access to the widest possible selection.

Also, you want someone who will work with you day after day, year after year, helping you solve problems as they crop up and keeping you informed of new improvements or brands. In other words, you want to find someone who will be there for you, someone you can turn to for help if your hearing aid goes on the fritz the day before an important meeting or if your hearing changes and you need to explore new solutions. You need someone who knows you and on whom you can depend, so make sure this person has a good business track record.

Don't buy a hearing aid just because the company has good advertising, it is the first one you saw that can be hidden by your hair, or for any other reason than the right one. After selecting an appropriate hearing aid from various brands, try out this hearing aid in the real world. Then discuss the good and bad points with your hearing aid dealer until you are both convinced that this is the very best you can do for now.

Just because Aunt Bea's hearing aid works wonderfully well for her does not mean it will work as well or will be at all suitable for you. By the same token, if your friend George was cured by a special operation or medication, then good for George. However, everyone is different just as every hearing loss is different, and what works for one person is seldom a true indication of what will work for another. Go through the steps; explore all possible answers. Then, if a hearing aid is your best bet, make an intelligent, deliberate choice based on the best information possible. Do not allow yourself to be pressured by sales pitches or won over by other people's successes. Learn from them, listen to their experiences. They may come up with options you had not discovered. Then go to your hearing aid dealer, audiologist, or doctor and check it out for yourself. But don't buy a hearing aid from someone you don't know or trust.

It's All Right to Take the Hearing Aid Off

Lots of people are not going to agree with this piece of advice, but in my experience, you need to take a rest from the buzzes, whistles, shrieks, and crackles. There are two schools of thought on this. One is that if you do not wear your hearing aid all of the time, then you will not learn to adjust to it. Well, that's all right as far as it goes. But my argument is that constantly listening to the noise generated by many of these electronic devices is annoying and tiring and results in fatigue. While a person does of course want to wear a hearing aid as much as he or she can, that person may reach a point at which leaving the hearing aid in, on full volume, may be so irritating and stressful that the person becomes fatigued and short tempered.

I have found that it is much better to turn the hearing aid down or take it off rather than continue to wear it and become anxious or overstressed. After all, a person does not need hearing aids to mow the lawn or re-cover a chair. A little bit of rest time can be just the ticket to restore my equilibrium. That way, when I need full volume for understanding someone, I will not be so tired. Instead, I will be calm and refreshed, which in turn will allow me to understand the speaker much better and to communicate more effectively.

Becoming an Explorer

Each of us is different. That is at once a source of delight and discouragement. I cannot tell you what specific steps you must take to communicate better, no more than you can tell me. But we can help each other to try out new ideas, to share experiences, and to listen to what others have learned. "Getting the words right" is such a small part of communicating. Just as life is what we bring to it, so is communicating with those around us. If we bring to it all of our senses, including our common sense and our senses of discovery, delight, and humor, we can succeed—perhaps not every day or with every person, but often enough to keep us encouraged, to keep us trying, to keep us in touch with the world.

Five

Taking Control and Letting Go

The processes of taking control and letting go are an ordinary part of our daily lives. We take control of many things—a conversation, a job, a project, a workshop, an office, a classroom, and our children. When communication becomes difficult, these processes no longer work smoothly. We are suddenly confronted with the necessity to figure out what is going wrong and to try to find new ways to take control of both ourselves and our environment. Sometimes we must teach ourselves to let go.

When we lose control of communication, of interaction with others, this causes a host of bewildering problems. How can we gain back some sense of control, when we so often cannot comprehend what is being said around us? And when is it sensible or necessary to let go, to decide that we must either give up control or to recognize that this is a situation in which we cannot or should not achieve it?

As my hearing dropped, I felt bogged down by anxiety, stress, confusion, and, eventually, fear. Taking control became more difficult, and it felt as if I were making demands. Letting go became an escape from situations that upset me.

Taking Control

Being away from a quiet, controlled environment poses special problems. When we are in a bank or a department or grocery store, the amount of background noise can overwhelm the best of electronic devices and leave us in the position of either turning the device way down or off, or otherwise putting up with disturbing noise. And the situation is aggravated if we have to converse with a clerk or teller. So what do we do? I have found that the best answer is to control the conversation. With some thought and planning, both the speaker and I are spared a great deal of distress.

Asking for Help

When I first noticed my hearing loss, I said nothing about it. In less than three years, when I could no longer manage by just pretending, I began to put my pride in my pocket and to say, "I wear hearing aids. Would you speak more slowly, please?" Gradually, I learned to say this at the beginning of each encounter. I tried to remember to smile and to get over feeling apologetic and embarrassed.

To my surprise, the responses to that announcement have run the gamut from a salesperson simply pointing a finger at the total on the cash register tape, to stories of a clerk's experience with deaf relatives or friends.

People often ask me, "Can you read lips?" I will say "Yes." I really don't read lips, I speechread—a skill I will be practicing for the rest of my life. I have learned that people who ask that question often want to continue talking with me. They will move their mouths carefully, project their voices, or make other creative efforts to help me understand. Often they tell me of someone they love who is having trouble with a hearing loss or with hearing aids. I tell them to take those complaints seriously—they are real and distressing. I also tell them that I had a great deal of help and that they too can learn to give comfort and help. They thank me, and I answer, "Thank *you*. You made me feel good, by talking in a way that I could understand you."

No Apologies Necessary

You have to remember that others will not remember your needs. This may seem strange, but it is true. No matter how many pieces of electronics you hang off your ears, no matter how many times you remind them, people will forget. You may tell a friend that you cannot hear him because of the heavy background noise, and everything will be fine. Then, a week later, you may meet that same friend under similar or even the same conditions, and he will start right in trying to talk to you. You will need to remind him that there is too much background noise and ask him to wait until you leave the kitchen, or get in off the street, or move inside your office. The problem is that people with normal hearing are used to shouting above the din, and they forget. Yes, even my family forgets. To this day, I have to remind them every now and then.

But you see, that is my job—to let others know what and when I can and cannot hear. It is their job to listen and meet my needs, as much as they can. And it is everyone's responsibility to do his or her job politely.

I have gradually come to realize that I need not feel apologetic or feel that I am making unnecessary demands on others. We all like to help each other. It makes us happy to do our good deed for the day. When I ask for help with a smile, the response is prompt. When I tell people how good they have made me feel because I was able to perform well in spite of my deafness (for now I am indeed deaf), they understand how important this is to me and show their pleasure.

The Bible says that the Lord loves a cheerful giver. I think the Lord must have a special love for the cheerful receiver. It is far more difficult to receive graciously than to give cheerfully. Yet, by doing so, we give double pleasure to others and to ourselves.

Everyday Transactions

Routine errands may become frightening hurdles when we cannot accurately interpret the speech of others. Shopping, banking, eating in restaurants, functioning in the workplace, meeting with professionals, such as your doctor or lawyer, can become so difficult that we may be overcome by anxiety. We depend on others more than we or they enjoy, give up too many activities, and retreat more and more. Trapped in a downward spiral, the less we do, the more we fear, and the more we fear, the less we are able or willing to try.

All of us, if we fight our discouragement and are patient with ourselves and others as we learn techniques, can gradually improve our communication. Each success encourages us, no matter how small. Everyday contact can make us feel connected to the world when we are discouraged. Often, on a "down" day, I will deliberately shoo myself out on an errand, just to give myself a lift.

Planning Ahead

When I go on errands to places like the post office or the bank, I write myself reminder notes and fill out forms in advance. As soon as it is my turn, I speak my piece. "Hi, I'm hard of hearing. Here's my deposit slip and endorsed checks. Thank you. And here's a check for cash. I'd like three twenties, two tens, four fives, and ten ones. Thank you. Good to see you."

Why are these transactions in stores, service stations, shops, and banks easy for me? In the first place, they are relatively simple ones. Now that I feel comfortable about saying, "I'm hard of hearing," and quickly state my needs, everyone is cooperative. In addition, I am in control. I am the customer buying services. I know what I need, what help I am seeking, and I feel free to ask questions. Any feelings of embarrassment come from within myself, not from the way others treat me.

If you need help in a store, it pays to think ahead before asking questions. Initiating the conversation puts you in control of the topic and limits the speaker's responses to a manageable few. So if you have a question to ask of the clerk, try to phrase the question so you get the best possible response, one that will enable you to understand the answer.

Getting the Right Answers

To get the right answers, I learned to ask the right questions. For insurance, I keep that small pad and pen handy in my purse or pocket. It is often quicker than asking for several repeats. I am even beginning to think before I ask a question—a real triumph for me.

What kind of question should I ask to get the answer that I not only need, but can understand? In a large department store, if I am not specific enough and ask, "where are the slacks, please?" I will get back a confusing string of statements and questions— "Women's slacks are on the third floor, juniors are on the fifth, budget in the basement."

That is a jumble of lip movements that means nothing to me. Better to go first to the store's directory, if I can find it, and read the possible locations. If I need to ask the clerk where something is, I try to be as specific as I can, saying something like, "I'm looking for slacks, junior sizes, good quality. I'm hard of hearing, so I need to see your mouth." If the clerk responds, "on the fourth floor," and I cannot tell the word *fourth* from *fifth*, I then hold up four fingers and raise my eyebrows to indicate a question. This has been very effective.

When I am ready to make a purchase, I assume the clerk will ask me, "cash or credit card?" I can tell by her mouth movements if I have guessed correctly, and have my card, cash, or checkbook at hand. If she has said something else, I can always ask, "Would you repeat that, please?"

When I need the assistance of clerks for longer transactions, the exchange of information is still predictable, provided I continue to phrase my questions for easy answers. If I ask, "I'd like a different color, same size. Do you have it?" I usually get only a handful of responses—"Yes, I'll get it." "No, I'm sorry." "No, but one of our other branches may have it. Do you want me to phone?" "No, but I have something similar. Can I show it to you?" If I am prepared to put together recognizable lip movements and the bits of noise coming into my aids, it is not difficult to decode the exchange.

For example, let's say I am in a grocery store and I need to find the canned salmon. If I ask the clerk, "Do you have any canned salmon?" he might reply (while looking at the fruit juice bottles he is pricing) "Aisle 17 next to the tuna fish." Now, that may not get me very far. If he did not look directly at me (which often happens), if he spoke quickly (which many people do), or if there was a lot of background noise (which there almost always is), I probably did not get much or any of his statement.

Since I cannot do anything about the background noise or the clerk's speech patterns, I concentrate on the response itself. I give the clerk a big smile and say, "I'm hard of hearing. Could you please *show* me where the canned salmon is? I can't seem to find it." Even the busiest clerks will at least point me to the correct aisle, and many will lead me right to what I am looking for. Or I might ask, "What aisle is the canned salmon on?" I can then watch for the number on the clerk's lips and repeat it back to be sure I understood. What I am doing is using the language to get the response that I need. The original question, "Do you have any canned salmon?" can be answered many different ways, including "yes" or "no." But a request for specific words or action commonly initiates a specific response.

Asking people to show you the items you are looking for, rather than asking where they are, may seem a bit demanding. You may feel that you are wasting the clerk's time, but this is really not so. It might take less time for the clerk to show you where an item is than to have a clerk repeat instructions several times. Most importantly, it is the clerk's job to help you successfully complete your shopping tasks. If you ask politely, with a smile and a thank you, most people will be happy to help you. And remember, the ones that are crabby are nasty to everyone, not just to hearing-impaired people.

This technique is not a trick or gimmick. I anticipate the situation and try to phrase my need or question as specifically and as clearly as I can, so that I can understand the response. Yes, this takes work, and no, the system is not perfect. I still have plenty of misunderstandings and slipups. But most of my daily interaction with strangers can be eased if I take control—both of the conversation by speaking first and of the responses by being as specific as I can or by phrasing questions in such a way that I get the response I need.

For every transaction, some kind of workable solution exists. That is only true, however, if I learn to take my mistakes in stride, figure out what went wrong, and try to do better the next time.

Meeting New People

Sometimes we learn by planning ahead, and other times we learn by doing.

Because boating is my husband Bill's primary interest outside of family and work, we belong to Portland Yacht Club, which is located on the Columbia River. At times, visitors from other states and countries come to visit our club. For years, Bill and I made it a habit, when we saw strangers looking about doubtfully, to introduce ourselves, to chat with them, and to help them if they needed it.

Bill's surgeries and my increasing deafness had kept us from attending the club's very informal Saturday lunches. But one day, in June 1985, we decided to go back. We entered and saw a young couple signing the club's guest book. Bill looked at me with a question in his eyes. Did I have the courage, he was silently asking me, to tackle strangers? My heart thumped hard. Was I going to change the lifetime habit of being kind to strangers because I was afraid I could not handle the realities of a hearing loss? Did doing what was right have anything to do with being comfortable? Shame battened down my fears, and I signaled with a quick nod of my head.

Controlling the Conversation

Dr. Donald Holden

If a person seizes control of a conversation in a careful, articulate manner and slows up the pace of the verbal exchange, the result will often be reduced confusion and a reduced level of noise. In group or social situations, taking control and reducing the number of people involved in a conversation from three or four to two can greatly increase the hearing-impaired person's understanding, ability to follow conversational ebbs and flows, and enjoyment.

We introduced ourselves, Bill carefully repeating their first names to me, and then we started toward the dining room. As we picked up meals, I wondered how on earth I was going to act as an effective hostess to this pleasant woman, in a room with bare wooden floors, full-length glass windows, metal chairs and tables, and the hullabaloo of conversational noise that creates one of the worst acoustical areas in Portland.

"I'm deaf, but I'll watch your mouth, and we'll do fine," I said and smiled at her as we sat down. "Just a second, while I fix my 'mechanical ears.'" I turned my cochlear implant processor up because it was capable of picking up a voice tone over the clatter, and turned my hearing aid down to keep my head from being blasted.

Now what? I wondered. *Questions,* I thought, *keep asking questions.* I pulled my ever ready pad and pen out of my purse, set it between the woman and myself, and began, "Where do you live?" She told me, but I missed it and asked her to write it down. If I was going to function at all, I needed some basic facts beyond her name. She wrote, "East of San Francisco, in a suburb along the Sacramento River." I knew this area, and was tempted to make some remarks about visiting our son Allen and his wife Elaine during his medical residency there, but reminded myself to stick to questions. "Do you like living there?" I asked. Her extensive descriptions of the area's pros and cons followed. I missed many of the details, but continued anyway. "Do you have special interests in your area?" "Do you have a boat?" "Where do you keep it?" "Where do you sail?"

Fortunately, she was an outgoing and vivacious person. When I missed a phrase or name that I guessed might be important, I asked her to write it down. It almost seemed to be working! As my fear and anxiety lessened, I understood a few more key words or phrases.

She seemed to sense my interest in her as a person. Realizing that we all love to talk about ourselves, but that some reciprocity is important, I inserted short remarks about our own lives, our children, and our sailing. I always ended each remark with a question to her. I was genuinely interested. But just as important, I was discovering a workable new technique.

If I took control of the conversation and asked the questions, I automatically knew the topic. I could listen, and even if I understood only a fraction of the words, I could guess enough to proceed with another question. Her enthusiasm and her attempts to help me understand added to our rapport.

Across the table, Bill and her husband had been having a lively conversation. Our lunch over, we rose from the table and expressed our delight in each others' company. As we parted, her final words to me were, "I've never enjoyed a conversation more. Thank you."

"Thank *you*," I responded, and in my heart I thought: Thank you for making me feel like a successful conversationalist when I needed it so badly. Thank you for teaching me a new technique that I can refine and use for the rest of my life. Thank you for being so sympathetic and delightful a person that we could make it work. Thank you for giving me back a small piece of the world I thought was gone forever.

I look back on that day not only as a happy milestone, but as a turning point. In one fell swoop, the scattered pieces of the lessons that Bill and Kay had taught me fell into place, like the pieces of a puzzle. The efforts of my brain and mind to make sense of speech and all the techniques I had learned became an arsenal of weapons I could use to fight for those missing words.

Appointments with Professionals

Learning to deal with people of the so-called professional classes has been, for me, a very difficult process. Yet, it is these very professionals—physicians and surgeons, building and mechanical contractors, lawyers, accountants and business people—from whom we need the most understanding and help. Sometimes we get it; sometimes we do not.

I have always felt that these people were above me, despite their graciousness to me. I feel, on visiting them, that they are very busy with important matters, and I must not take up their time. Bill has reminded me, over and over, that I am, after all, their client, and without clients, they would not be able to practice. It is up to me to make a permanent change in my viewpoint.

Nothing is to be gained, I keep reminding myself, by not taking a few necessary moments, at the beginning of a meeting, to move the office chairs to gain maximum lighting, to say that I must sit right next to a particular person and not be separated by the barrier of a large desk, and to explain and demonstrate the kind of speech habits I need from others in order to understand.

It is hard for most of us to ask professionals to change their ways on our behalf, especially in their territory. Offices of any kind are more intimidating than stores or service stations. We must make appointments ahead of time, either with secretaries or receptionists. We sit and wait in interior-decorated surroundings filled with "canned" music. And when we enter a private office, we are often shown to a seat facing windows while the professional sits behind that large desk. All these proclaim the status of the person with whom we must try to communicate. At worst, we are intimidated into doing nothing. At best, we tactfully rearrange chairs and ask for repetitions, written instructions, and slower speech. Our hard-won assertiveness is really put to the test. I keep telling myself, "You are paying for this person's time. You have the right to understand."

The speech habits of doctors, lawyers, and other professionals are no better or worse than those of the general population. Some mumble, some speak softly, some make enormous efforts in our behalf, and some simply cannot change their ways. When I have found myself dealing with those in that last category, I have had to make some quick decisions. For example, when I have to talk to a surgeon who is going to operate on my husband and possibly save his life, I ask him to draw a picture. That is a marvelous device, and I quickly supply the pen and paper. If I am speaking with a re-nowned professional, and I need help badly, I will find other means to communicate. (I write up all my information and questions ahead of time.) If possible, I get a family member or good friend to go with me to help clarify points and to ask questions. But, if this is a professional on whom I am going to have to depend year in and year out, and after several meetings, this individual is unable to modify his or her speech habits and behavior so that I can understand what's being said, then I will have to find someone else.

After I began to prepare for meetings by taking carefully written notes and lists of questions to appointments, my attitude began to change. Now at last I feel in control, sometimes more than in my hearing years. Now I enjoy watching the variety of responses. Some people are quick to suggest a quiet conference room or to pull two chairs together at a table in the office. Others are uncomfortable when I sit close to them instead of across their tables or desks. Their body movements of slight withdrawal and rigidity show that they feel their space has been invaded. I enjoy watching them gradually lose their stiffness, drop their professional armor, and display their humanity. Other barriers than physical ones have broken down. At my departure, when I thank them, their warmth tells me that it was also a pleasant change for them.

For Doctors Only

My regular doctors are so wonderful about speaking clearly and making sure I can see their mouths, that I did not realize at first how difficult communicating can be in small examining rooms. It took a trip to a new specialist to make me aware of just how great the problem was.

This new doctor talked too quickly and tried to give me instructions when he was behind me. I kept saying, "Please slow down so I can understand you," "I need to see your lips," "Can you talk a little louder, please?" Nothing changed him. His examination done, he mumbled his diagnosis at the same time as he wrote a prescription, with his head bent down, and his face hidden. As he handed me the slip of paper, I made one final attempt. "The acoustics in examining rooms are awful. Would you please repeat that slowly so that I can understand you?"

Impatiently, he stood up. I quickly rose to face him. He ripped out a brief sentence, turned and left, his voice still bouncing off the walls. No wiser than before, I was left bewildered, but also angry. I sought out and questioned his nurse until my information was complete, and my indignation was expressed and relieved. This was not what I was used to.

My regular doctors always wait until the exam is over before they talk to me. They talk slowly and carefully, write down instructions for me, and patiently repeat statements when I raise my eyebrows in a questioning way, until we are both sure that I have thoroughly understood.

However, doctors, just like anyone else, will not know how to communicate with you if you do not take control and tell them. The acoustics in examining or oral surgery rooms are invariably poor, and those bare surfaces and shiny pieces of equipment cause bouncing echoes that can turn electronically amplified speech to indistinguishable pops and squeals. You need to talk with the doctor and "organize" the examination. For example, if during the exam, you will have to remove your hearing aids, discuss with the doctor ahead of time what you will need to do, what questions or directions the doctor might have, and how you should respond. If you have trouble understanding your doctors even when they face you and you have your aids on, then tell them and also suggest that the visit start and end in an office, instead of an examining room.

Working out signals to replace speech is one way to overcome problems. It is vital if the doctor is wearing a mask or working behind your back. In either of these cases, you and your doctor can agree ahead of time on hand or touch signals to replace routine questions; for example, "When you tap me on the shoulder, I'll cough twice," "When you wiggle your fingers, I'll rinse out my mouth."

My dentist always lowers his face mask before giving me instructions or reassuring me. While he is working away, he creates signals with one hand to clue me in on what is going on, while continuing to work in my mouth with the other hand. It is all I can do to keep from laughing.

If the instructions are complicated and the doctor will not be facing you, another alternative is to have the nurse relay the doctor's requests or instructions. This may be a little more elaborate, but it could save time in the end if the examination is going to be a lengthy one. Sometimes the simplest, most straightforward way for doctors to communicate with me is for me to supply pens and paper for the doctor to write requests or instructions.

Doctor appointments are an excellent time for hearing-impaired patients to take control. I think you will find, as I did, that many doctors are caring people who will be eager and grateful to learn techniques that will help them communicate better. My regular doctors are never impatient with me, no matter how many times they repeat instructions or how many times they use pen and paper to write instructions that they would simply tell someone else.

Many doctors are ready and willing to be kind and considerate of people who suffer from a hearing loss. Unfortunately, some are not. You cannot change poor acoustics, but you can change doctors. If your doctor will not learn to communicate with you, find someone who will.

The same goes for *all* professionals. You pay them for their services. You have a right to expect them to do their best to communicate with you, provided you have done your best to communicate with them.

Talking to Children

I was baffled by children's high voices—their rapid speech when excited; their soft, quiet tones, and bent heads when tired, embarrassed, or telling me their special secrets. They often turned their faces away from me, causing me to miss their words.

Even more of a barrier was my own reluctance to tell them my needs. I did not want to sound like a scold or a nag, yet I wanted so badly to understand our grandchildren, our nieces and nephews, and the neighborhood youngsters who came to see us.

One winter day, a couple of years ago, I sat on our couch, fiddling with my fingers. I was scared. I still worried about whether I would understand our grandchildren, in spite of the fact that every time they had come to visit us over the past eight years, we had always managed together. But month by month, as my hearing deteriorated, I was always sure I would be "out of it" this time. The fact that I could still in 1986 function close up, face to face did not reassure me one bit.

Our son Allen, his wife Elaine, and their children Jacob and Amy were due to arrive at our house, after a five-hour drive from the Coos Bay area of southwestern Oregon. Our refrigerator and freezer were full of food, the children's books and games were in piles in the den, and their favorite stuffed animals were on their beds. Everything was prepared, except me.

It had been four months since we had last seen them; long enough, I thought, for Jake and Amy to forget to talk slowly with me . . . or perhaps just not want to make the effort any more. That was my real fear.

Jake had always instinctively understood what I could and could not do. When I took the two children on trips to the zoo, he always interpreted Amy for me and kept me in his line of sight when he ran ahead. As a small toddler, he explored my garden while I sat digging nearby. He never bothered to shout at me from a distance, but would catch my eye, make a gesture, and watch for me to nod or shake my head. He remembered to touch me when he unexpectedly came up behind me, and he developed a whole range of hand signals, both humorous and effective. If he saw me drying my hair, he knew I was totally deafened without my hearing aids. He would poke his head in the bathroom door, asking, "Can you hear me? Can you hear me?" I would give him our special answer, "I can see you, but I can't hear you." He would laugh and bounce away.

But would an eight-year-old boy be patient with me, interested in me? And Amy. I smiled to remember our earlier attempts at conversation.

"Amy reminds me of you, Ma," Allen said.

"Sure, she talks a blue streak all the time," I laughed. And she was no more going to slow down than I ever did, although Jacob had instinctively done so from the time he could first talk.

When Amy was four, I decided she was ready to learn how to speak so that I could understand her. Bill, Allen, and Jake had gone out to the boat, Elaine was off playing soccer, and Amy and I were drawing pictures and writing our names on large sheets of paper. "See, I can write Amy." She showed me, spelling the letters out loud as she wrote them. Then she said, "I have to go potty."

"Do you want me to come with you?"

"Yes, please."

She perched on the toilet seat, and I sat down on the floor beside her. I have her captured, I thought. Now is the time to show her what I need.

"Amy," I said, "you know I hear with these gadgets in my ears." I took them off and showed her. She nodded. "I can't understand what you say if I don't see your mouth. My ears don't hear everything clearly, the way yours do."

She looked solemnly at me. "Why not?"

"It happens to some people. Look, Amy." I brought the pencil and paper in my hand up to her lap. "Look at your name A M Y. AAAmmmeee. See it on my mouth. Watch me say it: 'AaaMmmEee.'"

I could see a spark in her eyes. "Look at my name, EeeeVvvv. See?" and I wrote it, and showed her my lips. "See, I can see the words on your mouth when you say them to me. If you move your mouth the way I'm doing, and talk slowly, that helps me to understand what you say."

She nodded her head and then began with exaggerated care to tell me what book she thought we should read when she had finished on the potty.

"That was great, Amy! I understood every word you said!" I gave her a big hug.

Suddenly she turned her head away, looked out the window, and said something in a plaintive voice.

"What did you say, Amy? I need to see your face."

"I said," she patiently explained, looking at me and mouthing her words, "that I wish I didn't have to look at you when I talk to you."

"Oh, Amy," I half laughed, half cried, "I wish you didn't have to, too!"

I smiled as I remembered that and wondered whether Amy had forgotten. After all, I forget all the time to be an example for others, even though I need their help desperately and I know I must set an example. How can I expect these children to remember after four months' absence?

The front door opened, and Amy came tiptoeing in, peeking around the room. I jumped up and hugged her. Jake was fast on her heels. In two seconds, we were back on the couch, one on each side of me, our arms around each other.

Jake looked up at me and said, "We . . . couldn't . . . leave . . . home . . . until . . . Mom . . . and . . . I . . . had . . . finished . . . our . . . soccer . . . games." He was solemnly moving his mouth with great care.

"Yes," Amy chimed in. "And . . . guess . . . what, . . . Grandma . . . Eve? I . . . have . . . a . . . horse!"

Obviously, they had been coached and reminded, on the long drive to our house, by Elaine and Allen. Bless my children. I hugged Jake and Amy to hide my wet eyes. "Would you like to go to the zoo tomorrow?"

"Oh, yes, please!"

What had I been worrying about, I wondered? Well, thousands of words were going to be spoken in the next busy days that I was certainly going to miss, and that was going to hurt. Sometimes I would look around in bewilderment at a suddenly empty house and wonder where everyone had gone, not having heard the quick exchanges of information.

Yet I knew that, at some quiet point in the day or night, Elaine would find me and tell me the latest news of their doings. I knew that while the children quietly watched cartoons on TV, Allen would sit at the breakfast table and tell me carefully and distinctly about his windsurfing, his hospital experiences, or the book he was reading. Everyone would listen patiently to our news and my feelings. And I could be sure that Bill would fill me in, when they left, on all he could remember.

There would be moments of wishing, aching, longing to be a part of the exciting hubbub. If I wallowed in those feelings, I would spoil their visit for myself. In time, they would notice, and I would put a damper on them, too. "Relax and enjoy them," I told myself.

Letting Go

Taking control allows us to get things done. But sometimes we just need to let go and to let conversations flow about us. At these times we must be sure in our own minds that we truly need a rest period and that we are not tuning out or avoiding situations because we are frustrated, embarrassed, or frightened.

All too often in past years, I struggled with discouragement, I told Bill I was reluctant to attend business appointments, conventions, cocktail parties, luncheons, or gatherings of any kind. Eventually, I even resisted inviting people to our home unless I knew them well.

This was not letting go. It was "ducking." By giving up, I was limiting our lives, increasing my feelings of isolation and helplessness, and accenting my resentment and fear. Bill was patient and sympathetic, but also persistent. He would say things like

—"You don't have to be the life of the party."

—"You need your friends."

—"I told them to come. You don't realize how welcome you make people feel. They'll understand. It will be okay."

And eventually it was.

Pretending and Adjusting

At first, when I was forced to let go because of my inability to keep track of conversations, I did a lot of pretending. My deliberately attentive face was hiding great surges of anger or self-pity, of resentment or isolation, and of grief over my losses. Perhaps that was hypocritical of me, but at least I was a part of the gathering. Gradually, I watched instead of listened, noticed instead of heard. I could adjust and adapt, or lose the whole ball of wax.

I do not see this as giving up. I have not picked up my toys and gone home. What I have done is to make a rational decision, based on knowledge of how much stress I can tolerate. With those I love, in relaxed surroundings, one to one, I can listen and decode for hours. My attention is fully engaged. When all is going happily, I can even forget my impairment. Love does work miracles. The effort still takes its toll, though. There are still limits. When I feel I have reached those limits, I let go.

Who's Bluffing?

In recent years, as public awareness of hearing impairment has increased, so have support groups. One day, I read about a new group meeting in a nearby hospital. I walked into a large conference room and took the only seat left in a circle of sixteen chairs. A short, young man standing next to a chalkboard smiled at me, introduced himself, and pointed to his name written on the chalkboard. I immediately noticed two problems: first, the chairs were placed in a circle (normally a good arrangement), but several of them, including mine, faced windows; second, the farthest distance between the chairs was more than fifteen feet.

The therapist asked the group a question. I understood one word, "Please . . ." Watching the people around me for clues as they nodded to each other, I caught the words, "Forty-Five Macadam Avenue." I finally realized they were stating their names and addresses. I took my turn, speaking distinctly, moving my face so everyone could see it.

The therapist smiled at me and said, "Welcome, Eve." Then he stood up, turned to the chalkboard, and wrote in large letters, "*NO BLUFFING!*"

I was stunned. Did he mean what I thought he meant? I looked around the circle. No one showed any surprise or concern.

"Any questions?" he asked.

"Yes." I raised my hand. "What exactly do you mean by 'No Bluffing'?"

He began to talk. I raised my hand again. "I'm sorry to interrupt you, but you'll have to speak even more carefully. I'm profoundly deaf."

"Okay," he said, exaggerating his speech. "'No bluffing' means that no one ever pretends to understand. We've all agreed to that in past meetings."

"Do you mean that whenever any of us misses a word or a phrase, that we should immediately stop the person who's talking?"

"Yes, always."

"Always?" I was more stunned than ever. "Not just here, but always, everywhere?" With my eyebrows raised in question marks, I looked at the faces around me. Now, they were no longer deadpan. Their eyes were alert, their mouths tipped up in tiny smiles, and their eyebrows raised back at me in amused recognition of a shared secret.

While the therapist was still vigorously nodding his head, I pulled out my mental "soap box," climbed on it, and began to speak passionately. "Do you realize what you are asking us to do? Do you have any idea how many words and sentences we miss in any ordinary conversation? Even here, where we are all being careful with each other."

I kept looking at the faces around me to be sure of their understanding and agreement. Every one of them was nodding. I took a big breath and slowed down for emphasis.

"If we interrupted others every time we missed a word or a comment, do you realize what would happen? Our family life would be shattered. We wouldn't have a friend left in the world. Oh, I'm not saying we should always bluff. Of course not. Not when we're talking one-to-one, or when we have a good chance of understanding. Not when it's comfortable to ask people to repeat or when it's important information that we need. You're absolutely right that we mustn't bluff then. But *always*? Ask the others." I swept my arm around the circle. Their nods were vigorous, and they chimed in with quick agreement.

Now it was the therapist's turn to be stunned. He settled down to learn more about this invisible, unimaginable condition called a *hearing impairment*. And we told him.

I have talked with other hearing-impaired adults and we all agree that, most of the time we are performing a balancing act. We teeter between wondering when we should stop a general conversation for our own sake and when we should smile and pretend (or bluff or let go). We seldom feel secure as the words run past us, as we receive too little information even to decide whether or not we should ask for clarification. We guess at the possible meaning of what we think we heard. We guess whether this is information we need to grasp, or not. Often we do not know if we have guessed wrong until we later bear the consequences.

Gradually, we build in techniques to steady us and make us feel more secure. In one-to-one conversation, arranged for maximum input, I never bluff. When I am talking with my family, a friend, a person who is exchanging important information with me, I try to pinpoint, as accurately as I can, what I missed, and ask for repeats as often as necessary. Some of my tried and true phrases are "Could you say that name again?" "I missed the last word," "Do you mind repeating what you just said?" "What address did you say? Let's write that down."

When I am in conversation with more than one person, even under the best conditions, I miss chunks of what others may be saying to each other. This is my loss, one I must face. If smiling and watching them is bluffing, then I do indeed bluff. I trust them to make a special effort to relay any remark they especially want me to understand. There are times when they remember my needs, and make extraordinary efforts for me. I am grateful then, and am quick to ask for a repeat, or a recap of the topic if I have lost the thread of the conversation. But I do not expect them to remember all the time. That would be impossible, especially when everyone else can follow with ease, and when they are all engaged in busy exchanges. I must let go.

In large groups or noisy surroundings, I bluff all the time. Anyone with even a slight hearing impairment does so. So do people with no impairment at all. After all, we all practice bluffing all the time. When we were caught daydreaming in math class, when we grew tired or bored, when our minds wandered, we all pretended we had heard.

"No bluffing"? You have got to be kidding.

Social Politeness

In social encounters, I remember Miss Manners' advice: "No sensible person tries to have a sensible conversation at a ball." We only go to one ball a year, but I have my own list of similar activities, and I apply the rule to cocktail parties, banquets, or any large gathering. A set of ready-made responses helps a lot to keep a grin on my face and my sense of humor operating. I might start a conversation by saying, "It's noisy in here, and I'm very hard of hearing. If I say something crazy or inappropriate, forgive me." Then we give it a whirl. Sometimes we even manage a brief, fairly intelligible, and pleasantly predictable exchange—"How are you? Did you take that trip? How was it?"—before I bog down, beg off with a laugh, thank my willing victim, and move on.

Surprisingly I have become a better mingler in large groups than I used to be. I have a ready out from getting stuck too long in a conversation—"I'm so sorry, the noise is drowning me. I'm going to look for a quieter spot and rest for a moment. I enjoyed talking with you." Then, I move on.

Noisy Places—Large Groups

In noisy or crowded places, people raise their voices and speak more distinctly. This automatic response makes communication easier for hard of hearing people, provided we observe lips and facial expression and that we do not expect too much. If I am caught by someone who, despite my warnings, wants to exchange more than mild pleasantries, my best ploy is to say, "really?" each time the person pauses for a response. It seems to cover a multitude of situations. As soon as I feel an opening (or closing!) might be appropriate, I make a gracious excuse and move on. I have no idea how many people I may have confused by this tactic, but it makes me feel I have done my best, and I relax and remember Miss Manners. On these occasions, being a people watcher is often much more fun than straining to carry on a conversation. I no longer feel self-conscious if I stand alone and look at people's faces, gestures, and maneuvers. Letting go is relaxing in these circumstances.

At banquets, I remark to those seated next to me, "Please don't worry about me. Chat with the people around the table. I'll enjoy watching all of you." Some people make efforts to clue me in. In that case, I bring out pad and pen for a little while and thank them for their thoughtfulness.

I remember one banquet in particular. Bill and I had flown to Southern California to attend a convention. While at the opening night, prebanquet cocktail party, a tall, beautiful, dark-haired woman approached us. Because of the noise all around me, I could not catch much of their conversation, but I missed very little of what happened.

She introduced herself to Bill, loudly exclaiming that they had a mutual friend, a well-known and much-loved member of the group. Since I knew the man she was discussing, I was ready to be friendly and to join the conversation, but I rapidly became wary. In the first place, she seemed to be making a big point about how close she was to our mutual friend. In the second place, she was totally ignoring me. Speaking in a voice loud enough for me to catch a word here and there, she bombarded poor Bill with torrents of rushing words. I could see Bill fidget and begin to look for an escape, but I just did not have enough confidence in myself or my abilities to interfere in this chaotic situation. I began to hit the panic button.

Then I stopped, took a deep breath, let go of understanding the words, and began to watch her. That cooled me down, and there was plenty to watch. Her eyes flicked around, checking to be sure others were overhearing her, and her hands waved dramatically to draw attention. She held her chin high, her shoulders back, as if announcing her own importance as she sang the praises of our friend. She was, I realized, trying to increase her own social standing by broadcasting and exaggerating her relationship to a person she viewed as superior to the rest of us. Although I felt sorry for Bill, I began to find humor in the situation. At that moment Bill caught my eye and noticed my grin of amusement. A smile lit his own eyes as he turned back to the woman, said something to her in his low, gentle timbre, took my arm, and steered us away from her. As we walked away, he leaned over, and mouthed very carefully, "I told her I had to go to the bathroom." As I dissolved into laughter, Bill sauntered in his sure, long-legged way toward the bar.

All of a sudden, I realized that I had caught only a few words, but had understood the whole conversation. Her actions had spoken more loudly than all those missing words.

I strolled through the crowd grinning, and ran smack into a charming stranger. This man handed me a delicious hot canape, introduced himself, and said, "I've been watching you. Does that little black box on your belt mean you are deaf?"

We launched into a delightful conversation. He spoke clearly and precisely and created openings in the conversation for me so that I could follow his thoughts and respond. I knew that he understood my problem, so I could relax and did not have to worry about making mistakes. We could laugh at them and move right along. The pleasant expression on his face, the interest and empathy we felt, made me forget my deafness.

After any busy or noisy gathering, I can count on Bill to tell me, later when we are alone, of any interesting speeches or any titillating gossip. It is just as satisfying second hand, and with all the boring parts left out.

To my amazement and amusement, the encounters that I used to dread have become among the easiest to deal with. Large social gatherings and conventions, traveling and functioning in strange and noisy environments, all now have carefully thought out solutions or limitations to which I have, to a large extent, adapted.

Tough Problems—Tough Decisions

The degree of difficulty we encounter in our daily lives will vary according to the type and extent of our hearing loss, with our occupation, and with our personal lifestyle.

In medium-sized gatherings, such as luncheons or dinners in restaurants with four to ten people, a party of six to thirty friends in someone's home, or picnics and sporting events, we are going to experience a host of problems and frustrations. We are likely to end up deciding, "That is the last time I am going to do that!"

At first, I lumped most of these activities together and was tempted to avoid them all. With the help of Bill, our family, and friends, I learned to analyze each occasion and anticipate what to expect.

Restaurants are a continuing problem for me and other hearing-impaired people. The larger the group, the more I let go and watch people's faces. My pad and pen are often used by others to write a special topic or an amusing comment for me.

Sport participation also takes adapting. Our carefree enjoyment is gone forever, unless we can let go of our embarrassment and our old habits, and then work at adapting to new ways of functioning. Offhand, I cannot think of many sports we cannot manage, if we are determined. Using eyes to replace ears, hand signals instead of shouts, the beat of rhythms instead of the melody of music, I can still go to Jazzercize® exercise class, sail, play softball or tennis, dance, hike and climb, dive, and swim. It is an odd feeling, swimming in total silence. In the cold waters of the majestic Columbia River Gorge, I use my eyes for safety and to enjoy the incredible beauty.

Informal get-togethers, such as picnics, potlucks, camping in groups, and some indoor and outdoor games, present a real challenge. We have to let go of much that used to make these activities fun for us. We have to change our ways of operating and watch out that we do not take charge as a means of control. No more will we enjoy the jokes bandied about, no more catch the snappy answers, no more understand the chatter floating around us at the picnic table and the stories told in the dark around a campfire. It hurts. If we allow the hurt to keep us from the activities we once enjoyed, then it is not the situation that is damaging us, it is ourselves. We have to let go of our past if we are going to keep our present and future intact. Easily said. It has taken me years to get there.

It is easier for me to function in very small groups of four people or fewer, if everyone is aware of my needs and the setting is ideal. When I am involved in the conversations that are my lifeline to the world, those one-to-one exchanges in good acoustical surroundings, I can even forget I am deaf. However, among four or more friends, it is difficult or impossible to understand the rapid flow of speech between people who know each other well or who are discussing topics of mutual interest. Unlike large, casual groups, where spoken exchanges are commonplace and more predictable, the topics here are varied and the language complex. When I am with such an intimate group, the problem is compounded because I care a great deal more about what I am missing. These situations cause me a great deal of distress.

Dozens of variables limit how much I pick up in these situations: acoustics and background noise; the care with which people speak and wait their turns; the type of assistive listening devices I am using; whether I am tired or fresh, relaxed or tense; what my expectations are; and how much is being asked of me. The list is endless.

Deciding When to Let Go

The crucial factor in deciding when to let go is how important the particular conversation or communication is to us. If we have to let go, what are the consequences to us? We need to give a great deal of thought to this and determine just what we should do. Should we ask that the conversation be slowed down for us because we feel it is important that we understand or let it flow around us and try to catch up later?

Every situation will be different, every decision difficult. Each of us needs to develop a consistent set of standards that will allow us to grasp the greatest possible amount of information, while at the same time, keeping us from constantly interrupting. This is not easy, but we have to keep trying.

When I am with a group of four to eight people, I often must let go. Even eight years ago, when my hearing loss was only 40 percent, I was often undone by small gatherings of family or friends who spoke quickly, overlapped each other, or spoke in soft voices or with careless pronunciation. I became upset, resentful, and often felt they were deliberately leaving me out. I gave up and sat in silent anger or distress.

Today, I know what to expect. So do my family and friends. I plunk my chair down into the middle of the group and stay alert. If one of them notices my puzzlement, I might get a quick aside ("The topic is such and such"). Everyone speaks more clearly around me these days, including me. Still, my deafness is so profound that I expect to miss most of what is being said. I let go of the hurt inside telling myself to relax and watch. I can stay with the conversation in mind and spirit, even if I do not understand most of the words. I smile when others laugh. Just the act of smiling makes me feel better.

Usually I have an opportunity, later in the day or week, to ask one of those present if they can remember parts of a conversation (for example, "I thought I heard Jake say he had a trail bike. Did I get that right?"). I prime the pump of recollection, and then I listen to the details.

One-to-one conversations are the lifeblood of my existence. The way I conduct them with my family and friends is different from the old days. No exchange of any length is casual, quick, or unplanned. We have had to let go of impromptu, spontaneous, or easy exchanges. We must first rearrange chairs so that I closely face my partner. Lighting, acoustics, careful speech, all these small things are automatically considered. We work hard. Nothing is easy any more, for any of us. We had to let that go, too. But we are still talking. And still listening.

Six

Naming Shadows

Hearing loss is a peculiar handicap. It is almost impossible for hearing people to imagine or imitate. We can close our eyes in weariness, or in sleep, or to blot out some horrible sight. We can grope around in the middle of a black night and get a terrifying idea of what it might be like to be blind. But our ears never close. We cannot imagine a world without sound. Even when we sleep, we can still hear. Our ears are always on guard, working to ensure our safety by warning us of noises around the corner, footsteps behind us, a siren in the distance, or a cry in the night.

When we lose our hearing, we lose our feeling of being in control of our lives. Even a moderate loss robs us of important messages and of understanding the thousands of words that keep us in contact with family, friends, strangers, and the world around us. We depend on others more than we want and fear for our relationships. We dread this isolation. We paste smiles on our faces and pretend we understand what is being said. Inside, we are anxious, discouraged, fearful, sad, or angry.

Each person's hearing loss is different. Each of us brings to our lifestyle a different and unique personality and a different cluster of long-standing attitudes and habits. Some of these work for us as we try to adjust, some against us. Only we, ourselves, can identify these patterns. Others in whom we trust can help us to identify them, but only we can use or discard them in favor of more effective behavior. It is our job to listen, to pay attention to ourselves, and to do the work.

It is difficult for me to write these words, for I feel that I have been lucky. Looking back, I can see that timing was on my side. Had I begun to lose my hearing ten years earlier, there would have been no effective hearing aids to help my nerve deafness until after I had gone through a long period of desperation. Had I suddenly gone profoundly deaf because of illness or accident, I would not have had the opportunity to learn from my family, Dr. Holden, and our friends. Dr. Black would not yet have brought the cochlear implant program to Portland's Good Samaritan Medical Center, and I would not have met Chief Audiologist Lavina Fowler just in time to ease my fears of total isolation.

As my hearing impairment has progressed, so has my understanding of my role in dealing with it. Often, the adjustments I needed to make in my emotions and behavior could not keep up with my physical loss. Besides, it takes time to adapt to new problems, to admit to and examine one's emotions, to see oneself objectively, to puzzle out what to do, and to learn new and more difficult ways to operate in the world.

Being individuals, the dynamics of relationships between ourselves and others are very different, yet flaws in our behavior or our relationships become exaggerated by our hearing impairment. Each of us has to discover our own ways to readjust our lives, as I have found out in the last fifteen years.

Over the last fifteen years, or so, I have had to make many changes in both my attitude and my methods of dealing with people. In the beginning I was very frustrated. When I was among groups of family or friends, mingling at a potluck or picnic, I strained to understand. As I missed the gist of the conversation and the point of the jokes, the frustration grew into resentment. I wondered why people did not speak more clearly so that I could understand and enjoy them. When Twink, Bob, Allen, Elaine, Jake, Amy, Kay, and David all gathered at our home at Thanksgiving, mingling and mixing, laughing one minute, deep in serious conversation the next, I ached inside. I felt left out, anguished, afraid. And when I grew discouraged and desperate, I knew I was in trouble.

I suspected that only if I looked at myself honestly, from the outside in, could I find ways to deal with my destructive feelings. It is hard to change. But we can learn to alter our behavior, if we try long enough and hard enough. If events catapult us into being uncomfortable or distressed enough with the way we function, we either adapt or go under.

I began by asking myself questions instead of reacting blindly to my distress. Why did my feeling of being left out among those I loved hurt so deeply? Why was it so hard for me to tell them I had a problem? Why did I feel so stupid? Why did it trouble me so to lose the thread of a conversation? Why did I keep my mouth uncharacteristically closed, lest I say something embarrassingly off the mark? Why did the words *deaf and dumb* keep ringing in my ears?

After a long struggle with my inner turmoil, I began to search with adult eyes for the child within me, seeking to understand why I felt like this, and what I might do about it.

I was born in Brooklyn, New York, the fifth of six children. We were a boisterous fun-loving group, and I remember basking in my family's approval, protectiveness, and love.

From the moment I walked the six blocks to our public school, I set high standards for myself. I worked hard to be an A student throughout all my years of schooling. As an adult, I expected perfection of myself in two important areas of my life—at home, I tried hard to be a perfect wife, mother, friend; at work, I tried just as hard always to be right. I argued away my errors by defending myself vigorously to others and, especially, to my inner self.

I am forever grateful for the self-confidence instilled in me by those who have loved me: my family in my youth, Bill throughout our marriage, and our family and friends. A good self-image is a gift beyond price. Yet mine was flawed by the need to be perfect and the need for perpetual approval and love.

When my hearing impairment drastically curtailed communication with those I loved, I ached in the pit of my stomach. The perfect little girl inside me prided herself on being loved and on knowing all the answers. But I was suddenly unable to understand the interplay of conversation among family and friends. I was confused and hurt by insufficient information, and I was confounded by my sense of failure. For the first time in my life, I lost confidence in my ability to be lovable and to be right. Then, I began to wonder what I could do about it.

Flaws That Hurt

For five years, I tried to hide my feelings of discomfort and discouragement. At first I denied them, even to myself. They did not fit my self-image. Soon these emotions engulfed me, but pride tied my tongue. The cheery face I presented to the world did not fool Bill, but my refusal to tell him my feelings certainly did. He imagined all sorts of reasons for my discontent and often blamed himself. When I finally poured out my tangled mess of emotions, Bill was relieved. So was I. Now we could set to work.

I began to learn how to change. When I am distressed, I listen to myself. I may not like what comes welling up from within, but if I leave my damaged emotions deep inside to gnaw holes in my inner self, they will destroy me.

I look at myself as honestly as I can, as I am today and as I was in the past. Knowing who I am helps me put a label on those secret flaws that once seemed too awful to admit and lets me talk about them with the people I trust.

Little by little, as we have searched and understood, my pride has taken its fall. I have learned to ask for help and to accept it. I have learned more tolerance and sympathy for others. My family and friends have noticed the change, far more than I thought they would. In return, I have been rewarded with laughter and sympathy and stimulating conversations.

Throughout my life I have defended myself vigorously, both against others and myself. When I made a mistake, I spent a lot of time convincing myself that I had, indeed, been in the right, while an inner voice whispered that I was wrong. With all that mental practice, I had become skillful at arguing unfairly, even when I knew better. I remember several incidents vividly.

After a particularly fierce argument with Kay, when she was fourteen, I read an article in *Good Housekeeping* about how to argue fairly. I triumphantly marched upstairs to Kay's bedroom and asked her to read the same article. She read through it quickly and handed it back to me, waiting.

"Let's try it, shall we?" I asked, with supreme confidence that she would soon mend her ways and our arguments would disappear like magic.

"Sure, Mom, I think that's a good idea," she responded.

I was surprised at her ready agreement to the rules listed in the article, particularly, "stick to the subject," "don't bring up any past grievances," "no personal attacks," "each person gets equal time," "once each has said everything that bears on the subject, stop," and "don't refer back to the subject afterwards, unless you have something constructive to offer."

Kay, however, knew exactly what she was agreeing to. It was I who was in for a long lesson. In the end, over a period of years, I did learn to change some of my tactics.

Even so, years later, Bill made one of those remarks I will always remember because it hit home. "I can't argue with you. You shift ground the minute you sense it's shaky, you talk fast and throw in half a dozen unrelated defenses, and you don't back down until it's too late. I give up."

As I became less and less able to understand what was said, I put myself in a no-win situation. My old tactics of switching topics, arguing to win instead of to understand, and listening only for fault and not for meaning worked against me. Not only was I not listening, not attempting to understand what a person was saying, but I was also working myself into "battle mode." My heightened emotional state interfered with my mind's ability to create meaning. I listened for words that were not going to be spoken and looked for meanings I was not going to find. And I made myself too busy to understand.

Final victory over myself came when I realized I had two contradictory needs: I could not bear to be at fault in my relationships with those I love and I had to be right.

Once I recognized what was getting in the way of my being able to understand the speech of my loved ones, I could begin to reject those feelings of superiority and substitute compassion and understanding. I learned to listen.

In the early years of my hearing loss, I often misunderstood the speech of others, and this created an overwhelming sense of inadequacy that caused me to retreat from human contact and, thus, to feel lonely and depressed. I always had thought of myself as quick-witted and intelligent, successful in school, work, and most personal relationships. My hearing impairment dealt a heavy blow to my pride and my self-image. Once I stopped laying all the blame on my hearing loss and took responsibility for my actions, my pride became an asset, and it propelled me to want to do better and to exert myself in more constructive ways.

Now I am too busy to be judgmental and compare myself to others. My hearing impairment makes me exert all my efforts toward understanding others. Gradually, over a great deal of time, my view of myself and of everyone else has changed. I am more comfortable with myself and with everyone around me.

In my efforts to rebuild my self-respect, I became much more ready to listen to Bill's offer of help. Instead of taking his suggestions as criticism and saying, "But, Bill . . ." in self-protection and defense, I kept my mouth shut, my hearing aids on full blast, and battled my inner voices. Eventually, the voices gave up the fight.

Pride had built a fence around me. If deafness robbed me of my props, it also knocked down my fences. I found myself more compassionate, more ready to reach out to others.

Knocking down pride did not compensate me for my deafness. But it freed me. And losing my pride, oddly enough, strengthened my self-esteem. It now rests on a firmer foundation.

Though patience is a virtue, I never possessed it. I was born impatient, impulsive, and impetuous. No matter how hard I tried, I could not slow down. I did everything at full speed. I trace this back to my childhood. My brothers and sisters and I were adventuresome. At our farm in the Catskill Mountains we climbed trees and mountains, dove off rocks into the swimming hole, sneaked out at night with flashlights to find nonexistent bears. I happily tagged along.

We ran up and down city streets, sang lustily, and talked our heads off. The family dinner table was alive with heated discussions on everything under the sun. We interrupted each other constantly, our voices rising above each other. Only Papa's calm voice stopped us. "Children," he would say, "what are you arguing about? Bring it down to a definition." Then he would distill our jumbled ideas into unarguable conclusions and fundamental themes, helping us to place them in perspective, exactly as Bill does for me today.

What I did not learn in my childhood was to talk slowly, to listen patiently, and not to interrupt, despite many requests to change. Bill patiently asked me for years not to interrupt him, although he wisely made no attempt to change my sloppy speech habits. He told me that my interruptions threw him off stride and upset him. When I continued, he began to point out how many times I had interrupted him in his last sentence. I would momentarily hold my tongue. It never lasted.

Necessity is the mother of invention and of change. As my hearing deteriorated, I found this habit of interrupting was getting me into deeper and deeper trouble. I could no longer be certain of exactly what I was interrupting. What was before an annoyance to others became a puzzlement, as I interrupted and spoke on a topic completely different from the one being discussed. That stopped me in my tracks. I could deal with being thought of as a person who interrupted, but not as someone who did not have the wits to keep up with a relatively straightforward conversation.

The more I sat back and patiently listened instead of interrupting with my own ideas, the more conversations blossomed. I found

I had more to talk about with others than I had thought, especially with Bill. Listening to Bill talking in carefully chosen words and phrases, logical progressions of sentences, and beautifully crafted paragraphs, I began to enjoy the process of his thoughts, as well as the content. I had always known our minds worked differently, as did our ways of expressing ourselves. In the past, I had been restless at the slow, deliberate way in which he framed his ideas. Now this is a lifesaver because he is easy to follow and understand.

I have begun to pay attention to what is going on inside my mind as I listen to Bill talk. I wait to marshall my ideas and to choose more exact words to fit my meanings. My jack-rabbit mind, which zigged and zagged across the straight path of Bill's logic, got in the way of effective communication. I am now able to keep a firmer rein on my tongue. I try to wait my turn, to stay on course.

Heaven help us, I have thought, if Bill had lost his hearing, instead of me. I am still lagging behind in my efforts to speak distinctly, with those precious pauses between phrases that I now need so desperately from others. I start a conversation with conscious pride in my beautiful pronunciation, but then I get caught up in the excitement of sharing ideas and feelings. My lifetime habits once again take over and my good intentions fly out the window. I am once again reminded of the demands I am making on others.

The other day I remarked to Bill, "It's a good thing I went deaf and not you. You'd have gone crazy with my fast and sloppy speech, my constant change of subject, my interruptions, long before I'd ever have learned to change my ways."

"No," he replied, "we'd have worked just as hard, and we'd have changed just the same. We'd have made it."

Facing One's Own Reaction to Hearing Loss

I write today from the viewpoint of profound deafness, but that does not mean that I minimize the wrenching adjustments that have to be made to mild or moderate hearing loss. At every stage of hearing loss, we all stumble into pitfalls that trigger a smorgasbord of negative feelings in each of us. Others will not understand these feelings unless we can describe them accurately and uncomplainingly. Before we can do this, we must battle not only an increasingly noisy and confusing external world, but also an increasing load of internal feelings about ourselves and others. I, myself, struggled at every stage of hearing loss, and I expect to struggle for the rest of my life. But, I also expect to be able to deal with the feelings that trouble me most.

Fear

Fear is certainly one of the worst of the damaging emotions, yet we speak of it so seldom. Books and articles about dealing with stress, anger, grief, and depression make their way into our homes and conversations. I see few books or articles about fear, and no one talks to me about or admits to being afraid. Is it a taboo subject in our culture? Do we equate fear with cowardice? If so, then we may be afraid of fear.

The only reference to fear I frequently read is the famous quotation from Franklin D. Roosevelt's 1932 inaugural address. This statement, "The only thing we have to fear is fear itself," was first found in ancient writings and has echoed down through the centuries, attesting to its basic truth. Unless we can get a handle on it, fear will cripple us and rob us of our will to action.

We who are hearing-impaired face an odd assortment of fears, and these fears can wreak havoc in our lives. Because I have struggled with my fear, and because it is so little discussed, I am going to recount how I have tried to deal with it.

I began by admitting my fears to myself at the simplest level. I faced the fact that I became afraid every time I had to talk to someone I did not see on a regular basis. For years, I did not know why I could not understand the person's speech for the first five minutes, yet could easily do so within ten. Once I realized and admitted that the fear of not being able to understand was clogging my brain, I could begin to tackle it.

The first tangible benefit of acknowledging this fear was that it became less intense and retreated sooner. Hand in hand with that came a second benefit. Unhampered by the befuddlement that fear induces, I was free to greet people with enthusiasm; I relaxed sooner and adjusted more quickly to their speech habits. This warmer atmosphere created by my welcoming smile helped me even more.

The third benefit was that I began to acknowledge my deeper fears. I began to ask myself, "What am I afraid of?" and I came up with the following answers—I am afraid of not understanding and of being left out or forsaken; I am afraid of ridicule; I am afraid that I will not have the courage to cope with new situations, to make new friends, to try out new activities, or to attempt new tasks and travels; I am afraid that others will not continue to make the effort to communicate with me; I am afraid of not being able to handle my own emotions and of becoming discouraged, lonely, depressed, and isolated.

In response, I challenge myself. I take off my processor and hearing aid and go about my day with the deadness of total silence pressing against my ears. I dare myself to panic. I grow accustomed to silence and familiar with fear. I refuse to let myself avoid any activity or event because I am afraid of missing words and losing confidence. I search my soul for other fears and realize that if I let my fears conquer me then I open a Pandora's box of all the bad feelings I have strived so hard to fight. These are battles I will never win completely. What matters is that I never completely lose.

Most of all, I am afraid of Bill dying, of living alone without his constant love and companionship, without his help and his interpretation of the world and people around me. I realize that after

Dispelling Fear

Dr. Donald Holden

One of the most crippling fears that people with a hearing impairment face is insecurity. A hearing-impaired person hears a great deal of commotion, many different sounds, without getting a sense of what it means. The person's enjoyment of music is gone, and this loss cannot be replaced. It diminishes the scope of life and separates one from other people. Hard of hearing and deaf people lose the sense of surround sound in all its aspects—the songs of birds, the chatter of children, the pealing of church bells, the notes of music, the warning of a siren, the whole tapestry of surround sound.

However, insecurity can be overcome with the use of hearing aids and other assistive devices (flashing lights on doorbells and alarm clocks, television caption decoders, and TTYs, for example) that help keep hearing-impaired people in touch with the world.

almost fifty intertwining years, living without him would tear me into so many pieces that the adjustment to new ways of communicating would be only one part of a much greater loss. I would have to learn to live all over again, in so many different ways.

Facing fear, analyzing it, sorting out the cluster of problems into separate elements, and then seeking ways to solve them, was of enormous help to me. It gave me a method of operating that I could then apply to other troublesome emotions.

This routine, so quickly and easily described, is extraordinarily hard to put into practice. The more frightening and prolonged the situation, the more threatened is our stability and ability to cope. To overcome fears, we must try to reach down deep inside to find strengths we never knew we had. And we must reach out to others who love us and lift us up.

Weary of self-improvement books, I worked on my method of operation and made more lists. I tried to name each miserable feeling as it occurred, saying to myself: "I feel left out," "I feel frustrated," "I feel like I'm jumping out of my skin," "I feel upset," "I feel hurt," "I'm mad," "I'm down in the dumps," and so on. I listened to my hearing-impaired friends and added their feelings to my growing list. A pattern appeared, which I then put into the following chart:

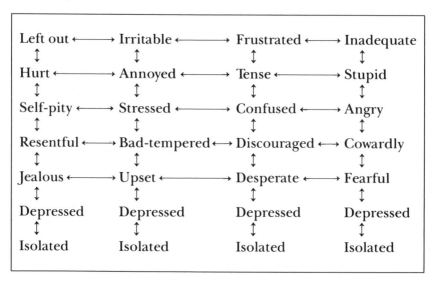

All these feelings interlock, and any one can set off another or all the others.

Searching for Solutions

Once I acknowledged my fears, I could figure out what to do about them. I no longer deny my feelings. I speak of them honestly, without dramatics or complaints, to myself and to my family, friends, counselor, or therapist. This puts me outside my feelings, even if only temporarily. We explore these feelings together, review past solutions, and brainstorm for new ones. I listen to others' suggestions, try them on for size. If I can laugh, I know I have made it, for this moment at least.

It all comes down to the fact that staying in touch with the world, for me, is an all-absorbing task. I cannot hold a conversation with someone and feel badly at the same time. I can either work at understanding, or think about how I feel. I cannot do both. Once I realized this, I knew I had to change my approach.

Now, I try to identify what is really troubling me in a particular circumstance. Then, I ask myself how I can best deal with it. When a new set of circumstances catches me unawares, I run through my list of techniques, to see if one fits. I may ask for help from anyone who is near at hand—family, friend, or even a stranger. Together, we brainstorm a new technique. If I find myself in a difficult situation, such as a free-for-all family conversation, or a large dinner party where I understand little, or a meeting with a self-centered person who is not going to make the adjustments necessary to communicate with me, no matter how carefully I explain my needs, I must sit back, let go, and deal with my loss as best I can.

"You can't argue with feelings," Allen once said to me. I remember that and let all my feelings rise to the surface of my consciousness. Then, I analyze how I am feeling—left out, frustrated, stressed, or angry. Sometimes the feeling vanishes quickly, once I have had a look at it. Just waiting it out may do the trick. Other times it becomes stronger as I acknowledge it, and I feel like wallowing in it for a while. No harm in that, I think, so long as I do not get mired down, or hurt myself or others as I stay down in the mud for a while. I know that eventually I will look up and see a better view.

If I bump head-on into an old, familiar enemy (and by now I have a trunk full of them), I have another trunk full of antidotes that often work—digging in the garden, walking or jogging around the neighborhood, running a short errand to chat with the store clerk, starting a new project, repeating a memorized poem or prayer, joining a new group, burying my nose in a book, thinking of every person I know whose affliction is worse than mine, and best of all, doing something nice for someone else.

A friend said to me recently, "Weren't you afraid to be a 'guinea pig,' to have that surgery and that cochlear implant inside your head?"

"No," I answered, "I was afraid not to."

Fear has its uses, and so do all other bad feelings. They push us to learn more, to strive more, to seek better answers, and to understand and love each other more fully. They are a part of our human condition.

Definitions: Who Am I Now?

"Have you accepted your loss of hearing?" a visiting audiologist asked me, during an interview.

I reacted with a quick, inner burst of anger. Greatly surprised at myself, and alarmed lest it show, I smiled and replied, "I suppose you could say that," and quickly introduced another topic.

On returning home, I wondered why I had become so angry. Acceptance is thought of as a positive virtue. It is the cornerstone of the Alcoholics Anonymous creed, which is so effective for those who embrace it. What was going on here?

Then I thought to myself, If I'd had only one leg, or if I were confined to a wheelchair and unable even to use my hands, or if I were blind, would a professional ask me if I had accepted my loss? I very much doubt it. I think it would be instantly recognized as an insult. So, I asked myself what word I would use. Immediately two words came to my mind: *adjust* and *adapt*. Yes, I thought to myself, those words really do seem right. But why? What is the difference?

Dragging out my *Webster's New World Dictionary*, I looked up the definitions of the three words.

"**Accept** 1. to take (what is offered or given); receive, especially willingly; 2. to receive favorably; 3. to agree or consent to . . ."

So *that*'s why that word made me angry, I thought. I certainly did not willingly receive my loss of hearing. I would have to enjoy self-pity or get a kick out of being dependent on others to begin to receive it favorably.

Back to the dictionary, I found,

"**Adjust** 1. to change so as to fit, conform, make suitable, etc. (to adjust oneself to new conditions) . . ."

This seemed closer to the truth. I turned back one page, and hit the jackpot.

"**Adapt** 1. to make fit or suitable by changing or adjusting 2. to adjust (oneself) to new or changed circumstances. Adapt implies a modification so as to suit new conditions and suggests flexibility."

That was exactly what I felt. Now I understood. When I am now asked if I accept my hearing loss, I have no emotional reaction. I am pleased that others are seeking to know more about hearing impairment.

With this increased objectivity, I began to think more deeply about these words and their significance to our lives. I added other words to my list, which serves as a guidepost to help me when I am discouraged. The list also moves me forward in my efforts to adapt, fight, struggle, learn, and practice.

I realized that my rejection of the word *accept* and my acceptance of the word *adapt* had strong undercurrents. I do not accept the fact that I can no longer understand the conversations of those I love so much. It is a loss. I grieve over this loss and seek substitutes, inadequate as they often seem. As with all losses and deaths, I try not to dwell on it. However, to deny it is to deny a part of myself and my love of others. If I accept my deafness, I may cease to find new ways to function, to learn and refine new techniques, and to practice and practice until these techniques become automatic. I will never, I vow to myself, *willingly receive* the results of my deafness. As long as I am able, I will fight for every gain that can be made, for myself and for all the others who struggle with a hearing impairment.

Getting Along with Others

In order to get along in this world, we must pay attention to other people's feelings and needs. Since I have to ask other people to pay special attention to my needs and my feelings, I realized I had to pay extra attention to theirs. Once I put behind me the thought that I would ever again function as a hearing person, I began to redefine my need for help. This need has become a daily part of my life and it will continue for the rest of my life.

How did I redefine my need for help? I started with changing my underlying attitudes and gradually altered the way I behave. Let me describe some of the changes.

1. I pay attention to others. I strain to understand every word, every nuance. I watch their eyes, eyebrows, shoulders, hands, bodies, as well as their mouths. I try to feel as they are feeling and to think their thoughts. Distorted as their words may sound to me, I often sense that I perceive their thoughts and feelings more clearly than in the past.

2. I am learning to accept help graciously. Fifteen years ago, when I first lost some hearing, I began to experience difficulty in understanding what was said behind my back, or through walls, or at a distance. In a burst of nobility, I once said to Bill, "This is my problem, not yours. So it's up to me to come to you, not you to me. It's my job to see that I'm in a position to understand you."

Had my hearing loss remained mild, that might have worked just fine. Many people with a mild-to-moderate loss that remains stable will keep in touch with their loved ones and in tune with the world by having a positive attitude and by wearing effective hearing aids. But this is not possible for many of us whose loss is more severe. As I lost more and more sound frequencies at an unusually rapid and alarming rate, it took every ounce of love, patience, and common sense that both Bill and I had stored in our reservoirs to keep up with the constant changes occurring in our life together. Without Bill's help, gentle teaching, and steady support, I would have become withdrawn, confused, and depressed. It is easy to find new ways to thank him for each thoughtful act.

Now I thank others, too, for the efforts they make for me. Often, when someone makes a special effort, a creative gesture, or a warm response, gratitude wells up in me. I tell them so and also tell them why I am grateful. For example, I say, "Thank you for using your hands when you described how you judged the horse show. That made it very real to me." or "You were speaking so distinctly that I understood every word. I even forgot I was deaf. What a boost!"

3. I keep working to improve my ability to decode speech. This helps others, and it helps me. I practice with my lipreading tapes and the lessons Bill and Kay have taught me. I try different adjustments on my hearing aid and on my cochlear implant processor's controls for volume and range, seeking maximum input in different surroundings. I remind myself that I cannot expect others to

work hard for me, if *I* do not work hard for myself and for them. This includes speaking carefully all the time.

4. I remind myself of something that Bill pointed out to me in 1985. Many people feel uncomfortable in dealing with someone who has a handicap. (If the word *handicap* troubles you, the hearing-impaired reader, I understand that. It used to trouble me, too. So substitute the phrase *person with a communication problem,* if you prefer. I preferred it and used it, until I became profoundly deaf.) People will feel uncomfortable in dealing with us largely because they do not know what to do or how to do it. This embarrasses and upsets them. It is easier to avoid us. I was truly stunned when Bill said this to me, and at first did not believe it. I do now, and act accordingly.

I now smile more quickly, reach out more readily, and inform others immediately of my needs. Saying "I'm hard of hearing" is often easier for people to deal with than if I am honest and say, "I'm deaf." With no explanation, that statement really stumps people. They do not know what to do. I have doubled their problem and their embarrassment. That is why I always add, "I need to see your mouth." Sometimes I add, "Don't worry. We'll do fine." or "If you talk the way I do, we'll manage beautifully." Usually such extras are not necessary, particularly if I give others early feedback on how well they are doing and express my pleasure and gratitude. It has been a long time since I worried about people avoiding me because I am profoundly hard of hearing.

One evening a number of years ago, Bill and I were watching a TV interview of Beverly Sills, the great opera singer. She was answering the questions with wit and style and with her characteristic enthusiasm and effervescence. Eventually the tough questions came. What of her daughter, Muffy, born severely hearing-impaired, never to hear the full glory of her mother's voice? How had she and her husband dealt with the tragedy of their autistic son, Bucky? What of the beautiful dream home they had just completed, only to have it burn to the ground? As she talked openly and frankly about these grievous events, the interviewer asked her, with awe in his voice, how she could keep smiling.

Her response went something like this:

> When I grew up in Brooklyn, my mother and I were very close. She encouraged me, helped me, and loved me. She thought I was perfect, so she seldom gave me advice, but when she did, I

listened. One time, when I was moaning and groaning over my problems, she said to me, "Bubbly, we can't always be happy. Happiness, and the things that happen to us, are beyond our control. But we *can* be cheerful."

I've never forgotten that. So—I'm cheerful!

When in the spring of 1985, Kay asked me to make three lists, she did more for me than help me to see my life from the outside in. Here are the lists, as I wrote them at that time.

1. Things I Can Still Do	2. Things I Can No Longer Do	3. Things I Might Learn to Do
Talk one-to-one in ideal surroundings	Understand speech in groups and conferences	Understand children
Understand TV & VCR, if closed captioned	Go to lectures and plays	Enter into structured group conversation
Watch my loved ones	Hear musical notes	Manage limited phone exchanges
Play games, swim, boat, and hike	Converse easily	Hear some speech in restaurants
Watch spectator sports	Hear doorbells, alarm clocks, and people calling me	Make new friends
Run, walk, and garden	Go on guided tours (can't hear presentation)	Speechread better
See, smell, and taste	Go to conventions	Use assistive listening devices
Drive vehicles	Participate in family conversations	Reach out more
Read and write	Have long telephone talks	

Those activities that I had listed under "Things I Can No Longer Do" began to challenge me. Could I truly not do any of these? That depended, I realized, as much on my attitude as my abilities. Whether or not I chose to participate in some of these activities was a matter of adjusting my expectations or increasing my efforts. I quite literally could go anywhere. The question was whether or not I wanted to and whether it was worth it to me and to others.

I can read plays, musical comedies, and even opera scripts in advance, enjoy the action on stage, and soak up the atmosphere. I now attend conventions and conferences, choosing a seat up front or in the middle of the room and using my assistive listening devices. I read rosters, agendas, and related materials ahead of time to familiarize myself with names and terms. I also ask for copies of written reports or minutes of meetings. After a meeting, participants seem to enjoy telling what they contributed to the meeting and what they thought about the other ideas presented. My questions signal to them that I am interested and involved, so that they are moved to make an effort toward me. I glean much from watching everyone, catching a word or phrase, viewing slides or visual presentations—and from talking one-to-one before, and after, large meetings in which I cannot interpret many words.

In time, all the activities I listed under "Things I Might Learn to Do" have moved to "Things I Can Still Do." In fact, that particular list of "Things I Can Still Do" is so long that I sometimes wonder at my discouragements. Yet, I am not kidding myself. There are moments when an unexpected upsurge of longing and loss engulf me. Little by little, I grow accustomed to these sweeping waves. They wash over me less often and with decreased force. They leave me undiminished.

Were I living alone and trying to thrust myself back into those activities that are now so difficult, I would pray that I would find others to help me and that my own willpower would somehow be equal to the task. I have been lucky. Others have needed me, as I have needed them. That is the best kind of helping, when we can give as well as receive. Because I have been so fortunate, I ache over the stories others tell me of their discouragements, their efforts, their stumbling blocks, and their determination.

For me, some real stumbling blocks remain. As I think of my losses, my throat catches. One is the loss of music. In the years when my hearing was dropping, Bill bought new and better stereo equipment. For a long time, with the sound turned up high, those Benny Goodman, Glenn Miller, and Tommy Dorsey records brought back the cherished memories of our youthful days. The symphonies and concertos by Beethoven, Brahms, and Mozart, which had filled my ears and lifted my heart since childhood, were still with me, even with notes missing. Now they are all gone. I will never again hear music—that heavenly sound that carries our hearts up to a special place above our heads. I cried on Bill's shoulder over that loss.

A far greater loss is the special communication that goes on when my family gathers. We are a talkative bunch, Bill and I, our offspring and their mates, and our grandchildren. The talk is peppered with tales of their doings, dry wit, clever turns of phrase, silly jokes, or fascinating ideas. I understand none of it. It goes by so fast, with voices interweaving and subjects changing, that I may catch a word here or there with no connections.

I have shed tears over this. Finally, when we were alone, I told each of them how I felt. Better late than never. Now, one by one, they will take me off in a corner and give me a carefully pronounced rundown on what is going on in their lives. Sometimes, one of the group will finish a joke, look at me, and repeat it carefully. Elaine and Allen have taught their children to speak with clarity and with pauses when they are alone with me.

Finally, after all the years of distress, I have learned a lesson. For all the hours when I do not understand their words, I watch their faces. After all, I ask myself, who among us ever really looks enough at those we love, or savors the moment as it occurs? So I watch their expressions and the interplay among them. I am with them in spirit.

I know how fortunate I am to have Bill patiently repeat for me the essence of what was said. No one can remember witty responses. The words are too wrapped up in the context and in the moment in which they were spoken. I have crossed that one off my list. No one can give me back those precious, free-for-all conversations that we all relish, and the warp and woof of family life. I have also crossed that one off my list. But as long as I have Bill to gather up the strands of a day's doings, to help me see the patterns that were woven, I am content.

What I will do without him, as the doctors and the odds tell me that one day I must? I have looked at that, too, and leave it to the future.

For now, I raise my eyes, and look at the people around me. I do not retreat. I stay connected to the world as best I can. I have learned really to look, to see what is real. The handicapped students from Grant High School come limping and staggering down the street past our house. I watch them. I help a blind woman cross the street. I see the others, some older but many younger than I, pushing their supports ahead of them as they inch down the supermarket aisles. I am grateful that my loss and my life allow me to see and read, to walk, run, or drive, and to be independent.

I remind myself that I can smile, hug, gesture, smell, taste, feel, and watch. Use your eyes, I tell myself. Can I ever savor deeply enough the beauty of the world around me, the sky above me, the birds fluttering in the trees? Have I looked often enough at the beloved faces around me with fresh eyes? I think not. I remember lines from a poem by Rupert Brooke, in which he describes his view of immortality:

> And [we can] feel, who have laid our groping hands away,
> And see, no longer blinded by our eyes.

Others with hearing impairments are not so fortunate. I think of Helen Keller and am in awe of what she achieved. I think of those who live alone, and worry about how they deal with loneliness, isolation, silence; how they find the knowledge and the help to do all those things that Bill and others have done for me. I think of those who have had no effective assistance in learning to use their hearing aids, or who are emotionally frustrated and physically exhausted by the harsh tones and mushy speech sounds. I think of the sick and the elderly who do not have the strength, the nimble fingers, or the healthy nervous systems to help them adjust to uncomfortable, new devices and sensations, and no one with the time or the information to encourage them.

I have stopped crying for myself. I haven't the time, anymore. I am too busy saying prayers for others.

Part Two
Language and the Mind

Introduction

Hello. My name is Kay Thomsett. If you started reading this book at the beginning, you know, by now, that I am Eve's youngest daughter. Eve has passed the baton to me, and I will assume the task of writing to you from here on out.

My mother has described to you that beautiful spring day she was sitting in the backyard amid the early flowers, crying. I had come to visit her and to talk about some ideas I had that might help her, but when I walked out the back door and saw her crying, everything I had wanted to say flew out of my head. It wasn't so much that she was crying. She and I have sat crying over a poem, a photograph, a movie. When we're touched emotionally, we cry. It was the way she was crying, her hands gripping the arms of the patio chair, her shoulders hunched, her face up, her eyes blind. She looked as if she were in deep mourning, helpless in fate's grip and in God's will.

I had closely watched Mom's descent into silence for two years, ever since my husband David and I had moved to Portland. I also watched my mother struggle to hang on to one more sound. She went to specialists for help—audiologists, surgeons, speech therapists, and speechreading teachers. I thought to myself that what I had learned about linguistics might help her, but in the face of these professionals I was afraid to try. "They must know what they are doing," I thought to myself, "I don't want to interfere with their methods, don't want to do any harm." Such thoughts bound me to inaction, until that day.

As I stood and watched my mother cry under a cobalt sky, surrounded by flowers and a loving family, my resolve stiffened. By God, I thought, I could not make it worse. So what if it might not work? So what if one of the people she was seeing might get annoyed or angry? She was my mother, and I had to try.

So I did. With what I knew about linguistics in hand, I hit the library for what I could not remember or did not know. I always felt that this knowledge would help, but neither Eve nor I could have imagined how much. Eve began to feel all right about getting tired and forgetting because she knew the reasons why it was happening. She began to head off stress and to increase her effective concentration time. Her ability to follow conversations improved, even though her hearing continued to deteriorate. Today, she has more social confidence than ever, something none of us ever dreamed was possible.

Was this a miracle? Not at all. It was the result of hard work. None of the information presented in the next four chapters will provide a "quick fix." Understanding the concepts introduced in these chapters and putting the suggested techniques into practice will probably be difficult. These linguistic skills will need to be practiced over and over, through the years, and the mental and linguistic barriers will always be present.

Why, then, include these chapters in this book? Because when all is said and done, these are the basics of understanding spoken communication. Just as a person cannot become a great chef without understanding how basic ingredients interact and affect other ingredients, a person would have a hard time overcoming difficulties in communication without understanding the process of communication. A person's hearing may deteriorate, hearing aids may improve, other people's speech habits can get better or worse, environments can change, but communication and the ways in which the brain and mind process it remain constant. These notions are the bedrock on which understanding rests.

The two major areas of communication that will be covered in the next four chapters are psycholinguistics and sociolinguistics. Psycholinguistics (psycho = mind; linguistics = language) is the study of the mind and language, that is, how language is transformed into thought, and thought into language. We will focus on three specific areas of psycholinguistics—prediction, sound, and memory (see chapters 7, 8, and 9). Attention will be directed to how the understanding of these areas of study can directly benefit hearing-impaired people and allow them to get more out of normal spoken communication. We will talk about how to work with the mind instead of against it, where panic comes from, why hearing-impaired people become so fatigued so quickly, and what you can do about these problems.

In chapter 10, we will look at another field of study—sociolinguistics (socio = society, linguistics = language). This is the study of how we use language in a social context to get things done, whether it be getting someone to open a window, making a newcomer feel welcome, or putting someone in his or her place. Too often we think of spoken language as just a way to move information from one person to another, but it is much more complex than that.

We use language to define our place in society and in turn to "place" others. We also use it as a defense, to fight, to make love, or to show compassion, anger, and sympathy; in other words, to express the whole gamut of human desires, needs, and emotions. A hearing impairment interferes with the ability to interpret these social signals. Hearing-impaired people not only miss the words, but also miss the emotional or social slant or the impact of those words. In chapter 10, we will examine the different levels of meaning in language and offer some suggestions for noticing the social aspects of spoken communication.

Eve and I based our choices of what to include in this section solely on the criteria of what seemed to help Eve the most. Both psycholinguistics and sociolinguistics are vast, complex fields of study, so we could not include everything. Although we probably left out material that could be helpful to someone, we stuck to what we consider to be the basics, those mental or linguistic operations that directly apply to the hearing-impaired person who is experiencing problems in understanding normal spoken communication.

We believe that before people can change the pattern of confusion and begin to restore some control over spoken communication, they must first understand the sources of confusion. This is the beginning place of that understanding.

Seven

Predicting Meaning

In this chapter we are going to explore a few of the methods our minds use to understand language, how language works to take advantage of those methods, and how our language is structured to help us gather meaning from conversation. Many researchers have produced an enormous amount of information on how meaning is made. The research in this chapter comes from a variety of sources, but my main source is Dr. William P. Costello, a noted researcher in the field of psycholinguistics. He not only introduced me to the world of language acquisition, but taught me to keep both of my feet firmly planted in reality. He reminded me that theory is wonderful, but if it does not work, if it does not help someone, then it is not worth a lot. The concepts presented in this chapter work. I would like to give you a brief glimpse into some of the things I have learned and how you can use these discoveries to your advantage.

Pinpoint the Topic

If you know the topic of a sentence or a conversation, then you can better piece together the meaning of words you might miss in a sentence. But more than that, understanding the topic is the first step in consciously using what the mind does naturally to enhance your understanding of the meaning of entire conversations.

The topic is sometimes a single word, like *Joanne* or *shopping*, but much more often it is a summary, such as *We are talking about Joanne, Mary, and Louise shopping at the White Stag skiwear sale.* When you know the topic, you really know two things. You know generally that the words used in the conversation will relate to clothes shopping, and you also know many of the specific nouns or subjects—*Joanne, Mary, Louise, White Stag, skiwear,* and *sale.*

When you know the topic, which includes many of the actual words that will be used, you are in an excellent position to follow the conversation. For example, the speaker might say, "Joanne bought a sweater at the White Stag skiwear sale today." You might hear:

> Joah bhhht-ah shhdhh at-thh hiidsstah-skiwhh-shh-tudhh. (the *h* stands for unstressed, indistinguishable sound) (Mackay, 1978).

With the summary in mind, our example sentence becomes easier to decode. We are listening for words that relate to shopping for a limited number of items. In fact, the only word a listener would probably need to understand is *sweater.* The listener could then guess, probably correctly, the meaning of the sentence (Howards, 1980).

Unless this listener is already clued in on the probable contents of a conversation, she is going to get discouraged and confused by the second word in the sentence. Without the topic and all the information it contains, the only word the listener might have a shot at is *Joanne.* If this is the first sentence of a conversation, the listener is in real trouble. In fact, the listener is caught between the proverbial "rock and a hard place." The listener cannot know the contents of a conversation until someone has started it, yet the listener will have the most trouble at the beginning of a conversation because he or she does not already know the topic.

This is why asking for the topic is so very important! Knowing the topic is fundamental to our understanding of spoken language regardless of the state of our hearing, but for the hearing-impaired person, knowing the topic is vital.

Prediction: The Art of Good Guessing

Once you know the topic, you know much more than just a few words that have already been spoken. In a way, you know what words are going to come next. Think about that: If you could guess with reasonable accuracy what words were going to be spoken next, how much better would your chances be of understanding them? Lots better.

To understand how this process works, we need to take a look at what the mind does when it decodes words and makes meaning. First of all, consider the difference between understanding something and memorizing something. Which do you do more often? When you memorize, you learn something word for word so you can repeat it exactly, the way an actor memorizes a script. But in daily life, we memorize very little. In fact, we usually memorize only things like short shopping lists or what we need to take to work with us on a given day. If our lists get very long (anything much beyond five to seven items), we tend to write them down (Smith, 1978).

When it comes to remembering exact words or items, most of us are not very good at it. However, we are very good at remembering ideas or general meaning. We remember that a friend of ours visited yesterday and what we talked about, but we tend not to remember the exact words our friend used or even the order in which we talked about things (Costello, 1981–1984).

The reason for this is, in a sense, we did not understand the words. Words are just vehicles for ideas, for pictures and concepts. We hear the words, then use what we know of their meaning to build pictures, ideas, or thoughts in our own words (Howards, 1980).

The speaker says the words, such as, "Joe hit Larry while they were eating at the corner cafe yesterday." Since we know what Joe and Larry look like and what the inside of a cafe looks like (even though we may never have been in this particular one before), we build a picture of Joe punching Larry in the jaw, of Larry going backwards into someone's hamburger and strawberry shake and landing on a black and white tile floor with a terrible crash! It is the picture, or the meaning behind the words, that we remember. After all, all our friend said was that Joe hit Larry. The listener imagined the punch in the jaw.

Our minds remember the meaning of the words and not the words themselves. You are really going against what the mind is trying to do when you try to remember each exact word the speaker is using. The mind does not care about the words themselves; it only wants to understand the meaning being carried by those words. The trick then becomes to encourage the mind to get meaning from the important words, and in order to do that, you need to become very good at predicting meaning.

Our minds predict meaning, or more exactly, guess what the person is going to say next. When we are listening to a conversation about a member of our family, we expect certain words to be used. Among these words would be the names of our brothers or sisters, or our children or grandchildren, words concerning their lives or work such as *school, homework, baseball game,* or *promotion,* and words concerning daily life such as *dinner, home, Mother's Day,* and *grocery shopping.* Once the speaker has started on a topic, he or she will generally be relating a story of some kind. Surprisingly, we can guess, with great accuracy, what will be coming next (Smith, 1978; Howards, 1988).

The Mechanics of Prediction

When the mind understands the topic of the conversation, it then tries to predict what the meaning of the next bit of information, the next sentence, will be. For example, if my dad starts a conversation with me by saying, "I had a call from your brother last night," my mind starts through a very predictable list of possible topics: how his wife Elaine did in the Boston Marathon; how their daughter Amy is doing; is their son Jacob playing baseball this summer and how is he doing in school; has Allen, my brother, bought a new sailboard? All this flits through my mind in a second, and because there are too many possibilities, I usually ask, "What did he have to say?" And then, guess what? Dad tells me how Elaine did in the marathon, how Jacob and Amy are, and how Allen and some friends are organizing a sailboarding expedition from Bandon to Gold Beach. It is all entirely predictable.

Most conversation is very predictable. You would probably think it was pretty strange if I suddenly wrote a sentence about the sabre-tooth tiger. While this is a perfectly good subject, it is not one you would expect to see in a chapter about prediction in a book for hard of hearing people. In fact, if I asked you to guess what words and/or ideas I would probably use in this chapter, I am sure that *sabre-tooth tiger* would not have been very high on your list (Smith, 1971).

When your mind is hard at work trying to understand a message, it is not listening to the individual words. What it is doing is more like this:

You hear the topic and understand it to be about a friend of yours. For example, the speaker might say, "I saw John the other day." At this point, your mind will build a picture of your friend John (as mine did when my dad mentioned hearing from my brother Allen). You will predict that the next sentence will have something to do with John, and you imagine what that might be.

Then your friend might say, "He said he was going away again this summer to his cabin." Since you know John well, you know he has a cabin and that he regularly goes to it. So far, your friend has said nothing you did not already know. All she did was confirm that John will vacation this year, as he has for many years, by going to his cabin. You might even have a mental picture of that cabin, either from seeing it yourself or from hearing John's description of it.

But you need to know when John will be gone because you are having a dinner party and you want to know when he would be free to come. So you ask, "Do you know when he's planning to leave?" Now you are predicting that your friend's answer is either going to be "No, I don't," or a date, such as, "He'll be leaving on July 15th and coming back around August 10th." If the answer is no, then the conversation moves on. But if the answer is a whole sentence, you will know you are probably getting the dates of John's vacation. You have predicted that the answer you are looking for will include the name of a month, and it will probably be a summer month. So you are listening for June, July, August, and numbers from one to thirty-one. The rest of the words around these important words will be words you do not need because you already know them, such as, "John will be at his cabin from ＿＿＿＿ to ＿＿＿＿" (Costello, 1982; Howards, 1980).

This is the way the mind builds meaning. It captures the topic, then guesses or imagines what the next bit of information might be. It then picks out those words that convey the information it wants and checks them against its guess. If it is right, it makes another guess, trying to imagine what the next chunk of meaning will be. If it is wrong, it revises its guess to what it thinks is right, then guesses again. Once again it checks to see if it guessed right. If it did indeed guess correctly this time, then it knows it is back on track and guesses again (Howards, 1980).

However, if the mind guesses wrong two or three times in a row, then it becomes very confused, and does not want to take in any more words until it is unconfused. At that point it feels as though all of a sudden you do not have the vaguest idea what your friend has been talking about for the last three sentences. When this happens to me I tend to feel blank, as if my mind went on vacation. This is the time you need to stop your friend and politely ask, "What's the topic, please?" Once you have the topic under control, you can begin to predict again, begin to understand the words again.

When your mind understands the topic and starts predicting, it is not listening to these words for the first time. All it is doing is matching the meaning of the words it hears to its prediction. This is why memorization is very difficult. Your mind is not really interested in remembering the words. That is not the way it works. It is trying to work out the meaning, and it does that through a series of steps, guessing at each new bit of meaning, and matching those guesses to the meanings of the words it understands (Costello, 1982; Howards, 1980).

When the mind hears a new word or group of words that it did not predict, it gets very upset because it is not doing its job. And its job is really very straightforward: It makes sense of our world for us and categorizes it so we can use the information to make predictions. Our mind works to imagine and predict so that we are not surprised by what we hear or by what occurs around us. This is a very important skill. By predicting, we can keep ourselves informed and safe. After all, you do not need to walk across the freeway to know that doing so is dangerous. You can predict that it is probably not the best thing in the world for you to do. Similarly, I can predict that if I call my sister "frog face," I will shortly be in great pain. After all, replies are not necessarily verbal (Abercrombie, 1968).

Linguistic Tools

The biggest building blocks to meaning are *topic* and *prediction*. Some of the tools that put these blocks together and make them useful to us are described below.

Structures and Meaning

Structures in language, the clauses and phrases, and even the ordering of the parts, play important roles. They bind the words together in predictable patterns and reveal relationships between words and ideas (Bornstein, 1977). Although very few of us can diagram a sentence (or would even want to), our minds carry an imprint of the grammar, or structure, of our language. The mind learns to expect certain types of words in certain structures (Soames and Perlmutter, 1979).

To illustrate this, let's go back to the sentence about the skiwear sale (Joanne bought a sweater at the White Stag skiwear sale today).

The listener knows the topic (Joanne, Mary, and Louise shopping at the White Stag skiwear sale today) and knows the structures of American English. She was able to reconstruct the first word as *Joanne* and the seventh, eighth, and ninth words (because she heard a one or two syllable word) as *White Stag skiwear*. The listener knows about the sale, so even though the next word is unintelligible, it is duplicate information and not really needed. What our listener wants to know is what about Joanne?

The listener has quite a bit of information to work with. She knows that *Joanne* is probably the subject and that the next word is probably a verb. She knows this because the most common English sentence pattern is subject + verb and because of the structural clues in the sentence (Robinson, 1983; Bornstein, 1977). She is trying to construct a sentence out of *Joanne* + verb + a "something."

The listener puts this together with the topic—the ladies were at a skiwear sale—and then begins to guess at what a person can do at a clothing sale. She can buy a "something," try on a "something," return a "something," or look at a "something." There are probably other things, but these cover the most likely options. Now, which of these would be the most probable? Would you return a piece of clothing during a sale? Yes, but not likely. You would try on and look at clothes, but something is wrong with those choices.

Looking at the pattern again, we see that the verb we are trying to guess is a one syllable word. Unless our listener misheard the word completely, she probably heard only one syllable. *Try on* and *look at* are definitely two syllables. The most likely answer, in this case, is the correct answer—buy or bought. So, Joanne bought a "something."

Before you throw your hands up and declare, "Heavens! I couldn't possibly do this every time," remember this: You are already doing it. If you know the topic, your mind is rapidly running through the possibilities, so quickly you do not even realize it is happening (Smith, 1971).

The result might be that you will ask, "Did Joanne buy something?" In this way you are checking your guess (that the verb was *buy* or *bought*) as well as filling in the missing information (what was bought). This bit of mental computing is so natural that everyone uses it to catch up on parts of conversations they miss. By knowing the topic and putting together the structural and meaning clues, our minds have a very good idea of what should come next. We can take advantage of this knowledge and ability by making sure we have what we need, which is the topic (Lyons, 1977; Howards, 1980).

Repetition

Claude Shannon in 1948 published a theory of information in the *Bell System Technical Journal*. He created a mathematical model of a message, which researchers could use to understand just how much meaning in a message got transferred from point A to point B. And after all, isn't this the purpose of communication—to get meaning from a speaker and give meaning back?

Part of Shannon's research focused on how redundancy (or repetitiveness) of language helps eliminate error (Campbell, 1982). For example, we take for granted the fact that sentences have subjects and verbs. What we do not notice is how we constantly repeat words over and over in our conversations (Robinson, 1983; Jacobs and Rosenbaum, 1971). Why do we do this? Why don't we just say the subject once and then not mention it again until we change it? After all, if we say or write it once, the listener or reader should remember, right? Let's examine this by reading a short paragraph on one topic that uses the subject only once:

> On a hot summer afternoon, my cat Crystal went looking for a shady, cool spot. Walked toward the bushes, but was frightened off by a woman on the way to the laundry. Sauntered to a stairwell only to be chased off by a puppy. Next, tried climbing a tree, but once up in the branches, couldn't find a comfortable place to lay down. Ended up thoroughly disgusted with the situation, came into the apartment, slithered under the bed, and went to sleep.

As you can see, we are accustomed to having the subject repeated for us at the beginning of every sentence, even if that subject is a pronoun like *she*. Here is the paragraph rewritten with the original subjects put back in.

On a hot summer afternoon, my cat Crystal went looking for a shady, cool spot. *Crystal* walked toward the bushes, but *she* was frightened off by a woman on the way to the laundry. *She* sauntered to a stairwell, only to be chased off by a puppy. Next, *Crystal* tried climbing a tree, but once *she* was up in the branches, *she* couldn't find a comfortable place to lay down. *Crystal* ended up thoroughly disgusted with the situation, came into the apartment, slithered under the bed, and went to sleep.

Repetition is another structural tool that clues us into what is coming next. In the above example, the subject was always followed by a verb, but not just any verb. All the verbs relate actions that can apply to the subject, my cat. This repetition can be used as a prediction tool, but it is more than that. It allows our minds to skip over some words and concentrate more fully on others (Chomsky, 1968; Soames and Perlmutter, 1979).

Carefully read some memorable speeches. One thing that many speeches have in common is that they are highly repetitive. Excellent examples are found in Martin Luther King's "I Have a Dream" speech and the line from John F. Kennedy's inaugural address: "Ask not what your country can do for you; ask what you can do for your country." Except for *not,* every word is repeated. Every structure is repeated, too. The phrase is in itself a two-part construction (called a correlative); each part echoes the other. Each half contains a clause starting with *what,* an identical two-part verb, and a prepositional phrase starting with the same preposition, *for.*

Repeating structures (and words) create rhythms that our minds first recognize, then remember, then anticipate. The differences in those repetitions, words, or structures stand out. In the hands of skilled writers, they seem to shine and sing (Robinson, 1981–1983).

Even everyday language is built to be repetitive. The subjects, verbs, and objects, and the phrases and clauses repeat over and over again, repeating the message. The reason is that language is very difficult and getting a message from point A to point B in the best of circumstances is often a risky, "hit or miss" proposition.

Listening for Meaning

The repetitiveness in language is one reason you can predict what is going to be said next. It is the structure of the language that lets you know when a sentence or statement has ended and when another is going to begin. The repetitiveness lets you ignore many words and still get the meaning of what is being said. For example, the following sentence is missing many of the structural words, but see if you can fill in the meaning.

___ ___ ship sailed ___ ___ world, ___ docked ___ San Francisco.

Remember, do not try to duplicate or guess at which words were left out; guess only at the general meaning of the sentence. You can take a clue from the punctuation (the comma, in this case) because when this sentence is spoken, the comma would become a pause. So what have you got? The topic is a ship. This ship did two things—it sailed and docked. If you guessed that it docked in San Francisco, you are right! Now take a look at the first part of the sentence and ask yourself, Where did the ship sail? Well, it had something to do with *world*. It could be *around the world*, which would be logical since a ship cannot very well sail *toward the world*. The fifth blank could be filled with *then, and, but,* or other words that have a similar meaning, so it really does not matter what the exact word is. The first and fourth blanks can be filled with an article, either *a, an,* or *the*. The second blank probably describes the ship, so it needs an adjective such as *tall, small,* or *sailing*. But does it really matter? Do you really need to know those words to understand the basic message? The answer is, No, you do not.

It is the repetition of the words and structures that allows people with normal hearing to be lazy and listen when they feel like it, rather than paying close attention to all that is said (Smith, 1971). It also allows people with a hearing loss to hope that they can still, to some extent, get the speaker's message.

My mother found that as her hearing loss became more and more severe, she began straining to hear more. What she was trying to hear was not more message, but more words. This led her into a terrible trap: As she heard less and less, she became less and less sure that she was listening for and understanding the right words, the words that carry the message. As an example, let's look at the sample sentence again, only this time we'll leave out the key words.

The tall ___ _____ around the ___, and ___ in _____.

Most of your guesses were probably right. But even if they were not, it did not really matter. You got the meaning, which is all that is important. Unfortunately, these words also are the easiest to guess simply because they are, for the most part, repetitive, structural words. These were the words my mother was straining to get, the very words that do not really matter. In the first example, I left out six words, and in the second, five (if you count San Francisco as one word). Yet, given only the second example, it would be almost impossible for anyone to guess the meaning of the sentence. The point is that the number of words you get is not as important as the usefulness of those words (Costello, 1982; Smith, 1971).

Hearing all the words is not the answer. In the first place, it becomes nearly impossible if your hearing loss is severe. And in the second place, even if you could hear and understand all the words, you probably would not. People with normal hearing tend to listen just enough to get the message, and no more. So part of the answer is to relax and not try to hear every word. If you know the topic and listen for the message, your mind will have a better chance of putting together more of the structures and words into meaningful bits of information (Smith, 1978).

Practice, Practice, Practice

Now that we have covered the pieces, it's time to put them together. Repetition is built into the language. You don't have to do anything to make it happen. Once you know the topic, the words within the topic will be repeated over and over, perhaps as pronouns (*he, she, I, us, them,* etc.), perhaps as proper nouns (*Peter, cabin, White Stag, skiwear,* etc.).

Structures and meaning will help dictate what new words you will hear and the order the words will come in. If the subject is a family camping trip, then the words coming up will most probably have to do with camping—tent, hiking, fishing, campfire. Knowing the structures lets us be even more specific. Given a certain subject, such as *rain*, within a certain topic (family camping trip), and given that a verb usually follows the subject, you will probably hear *fell, held off, came down in buckets, drizzled, soaked everything,* during the course of the conversation because these are all verbs that can be paired with the subject, *rain*.

All of the mind's guesses and ways of guessing together become *prediction*. But the one piece of the puzzle that prediction hangs on is *knowing the topic*. The mind will do the rest automatically if it has the topic. After all, if a person does not know the topic, any word can follow. The choices are so numerous that the mind cannot begin to guess what might come next, it cannot predict without that vital, first clue.

Getting that first clue is in your hands. You can ask for the topic any time you wish. As Eve pointed out in chapter 5, sometimes you may choose to let go; other times you will need to take control. This is up to you. But when you decide to take control, the first, second, and third most important actions you can take are get the topic, get the topic, and get the topic.

Sometimes the topic is created by the situation. These cases present a wonderful opportunity to practice prediction. By making prediction a more conscious act, you can begin to use prediction to understand conversations better. Remember, you already use it unconsciously; you are using it right now, even as you read. But, if you can make prediction a conscious effort, you will improve your comprehension of conversations a great deal and get more meaning from the speaker's words.

By concentrating on prediction, you will be more likely to hear and understand the important words because you will be anticipating them, not letting them come up and surprise you. You also will realize sooner when you have lost the thread of a conversation or have gotten off the topic. Then you can climb back in quicker, which can be critical if you are engaged in a three- or four-way conversation. You will lose much less time being confused and will start picking up the meaning of the conversation that much more quickly (Costello, 1982; Smith, 1978).

But how does one go about practicing prediction? Very simply, by thinking about it and trying to do it more often. Look at the following example of how you can turn a mundane chore into a prediction exercise.

Imagine you have been shopping in a grocery store and have taken your purchases to the checkout counter. In this situation, you can predict that the checker will probably say something to you. When and how he does address you will clue you in to the meaning of what he says. For example, if the checker says something while partially looking at you and partially looking at the groceries he is checking, he probably said something like, "Hi, how are you today?" If the weather is particularly beautiful, he also might have said, "Lovely weather we're having." And that is about it. He is probably not going to say, "I gave my son a new bike for Christmas," or "I'm in line for a new management position if I can just finish a class I'm taking at the community college." While both of those sentences are perfectly reasonable in other situations, they are not reasonable at the checkout counter of your local supermarket.

If the checker stops checking your groceries and holds up a can of soup, turns it this way and that, and says something to you, he is probably saying, "Do you remember the price of this soup?" And then, like most people, you would reply, "No, I don't know how much it is."

After your groceries have been bagged and you have paid the checker, he may make another statement. In all probability it will be "Have a good day," or "Thank you." If you have lots of bags, and especially if you are a woman, and definitely if you are a pregnant woman, he might ask you, "Would you like someone to help you with your groceries?"

Many people fear most day-to-day conversations with strangers. In reality, the topics of these conversations and the words most likely to be used are dictated by the situation, and, therefore, they are highly predictable. Conversations with grocery clerks will center around food, its location, and price. Conversations with bank tellers will be full of words about money. Another advantage of practicing prediction in these surroundings is that if you make a mistake, the environments are usually so noisy and busy (the grocery store, the bank, the department store, the gas station, or the garage) that any misunderstanding is instantly forgiven.

The point is that at any given time in any given conversation with any given set of persons, you can reasonably predict what is going to be said. The situation you are in, the person you are talking to, and the topic you have chosen to talk about will all conspire to reduce the number of possible words or ideas that will be spoken.

Researchers have varied opinions on how many different words the average person uses in normal everyday conversation. Let's say, for the sake of argument, that there are 10,000. One would think this means that the next word could be any one of 10,000 words. But that is just not so. Just as you do not expect me to use the words *sabre-tooth tiger*, you would expect me to use *hearing* or *language*. Every time I start to say something, every time I start a topic or a sentence, the number of words I can use next will diminish. For example, if I choose the subject or topic *diesel locomotive*, I cannot use the verbs *swam*, *loved*, or *wrote* because a locomotive cannot swim, love, or write. I can only choose a verb that describes what a locomotive can do or be such as *crashed*, *arrived*, or *was late* (Robinson, 1981–1983; Smith, 1971).

When you know the topic and are better at using prediction to guess the meaning of the next words the speaker might say, you should find it much easier to understand the words that carry meaning. For example, suppose you were back in the conversation with your friend about your mutual friend John, and you heard "faa-k-sh'n" and "k-b'n." If you were predicting the answer to be something about John's summer plans, you could better reconstruct the words *vacation* and *cabin* than if you had no idea what the topic was or what the speaker might be talking about.

Prediction gives you a leg up, so to speak, on the meaning or possible meaning of important words that could be spoken in a conversation. It makes it easier for you to take what you hear and reconstruct it into the words that carry the meaning.

Making Prediction Work for You

Prediction works on two levels of understanding at once. It allows you to become better at guessing the important words, and it keeps the meaning in a conversation flowing between you and the speaker. Even losing the thread of the topic is meaningful, for if the loss is quickly realized, you can stop the speaker and have him or her repeat or rephrase the current topic. This gets you back on track quickly and with much less frustration and misunderstanding on both sides of the conversation.

So it comes down to this: relax, get the topic, and predict. You do not need to worry about getting all the words. You do not even need to hear the words absolutely correctly. Just getting close will do because you do not remember the words anyway, only the meaning being carried by them. Work on making prediction a conscious skill, one that you can call on repeatedly and at will, to help you better use the sounds you are getting.

In order to become better at predicting, all you need to do is practice. You have the ability to do it fairly well right now because your mind does it all the time. What you must do is try to improve.

All you have to do to get better is practice during your daily conversations.

You might practice on a friend. Explain to your friend that you are trying to learn to be a more accurate listener through two methods—trying to predict what the speaker is going to say next, and controlling the topic by initiating questions or asking the speaker to rephrase something already said. Then do it!

Another way to practice prediction skills is to imagine a situation (such as our grocery store scene) just before taking part in that activity. Imagine what the clerk or bank teller or bus driver might say or do if you say, "good morning!" or say nothing at all and just smile when they say, "hello." Then watch carefully and see if you predicted correctly.

Eight

Rethinking Sound

In this chapter we will explore the relationship between the brain and mind. Each plays a unique role in our understanding of language, and each can be encouraged to do its job better. Before we begin, we must define *brain* and *mind*.

The brain is an organ of the body that gathers up messages and sends out signals. It does this through a very complex system of nerves and sensory organs that monitor our internal well-being and receive information from the world.

The mind cannot be described in any physical sense. The mind is the seat of thought, and it organizes the impulses the brain receives into recognizable patterns that can be utilized to form thoughts and progressions of thoughts.

For example, when our eyes see the word *cat,* a signal is flashed along the optic nerves into the brain. The signal *cat* is recognized by the mind as language, as something to be read. If the mind does not know English, it might not get any further than that. But if the mind does understand English, it understands that this signal is a representation of an animal. And, since most of us have seen a domestic cat, our minds make a further connection between *cat* and a small, furry, domestic creature (Britton, 1970; Vygotsky, 1962).

But the mind can and often does go much further. People who own cats, or have been fond of a particular cat, will think of their cat, remember its name, the funny things it likes to do, the way it smells, where it likes to sleep, and how its fur feels when petted. They will remember, in flashes, a whole catalogue of information about their particular cat (Chomsky, 1968).

The brain receives signals from the body and its senses, and the mind interprets the signals. The mind then keeps track of those interpretations and organizes them so we can remember them. In this way, the brain and the mind work together, simultaneously, to create intelligence (Vygotsky, 1962).

Too often the brain and the mind are thought of and treated as one unit, when really they should be dealt with as two separate elements of one whole. You must have a brain in order to have a mind, but a brain without a mind would not be much use to you. You need them both. Since the brain and the mind are inherently different, they can have different capabilities, limitations, and problems.

The brain constantly processes all the signals it gets from the body. When those signals are damaged or diminished, the mind cannot interpret them, so it gets upset. As a result, we can feel stressed, nervous, and irritable. Sometimes, we get headaches (Howards, 1980; Shaughnessy, 1977). I always know when I need a new pair of glasses because at the end of the day I tend to get headaches right above my eyebrows from eye strain. This is how my brain tells me it is straining to do its job.

The mind works very hard to make sense of the signals it receives. In the case of hearing, the mind must interpret sounds received by the brain. If the sounds are faint or distorted, the whole message does not get through. The cause of the problem could be hearing loss, tinnitus, or interference from high-powered hearing aids. The result is that some parts of the message get through slightly changed, other parts get through completely changed, and still other parts do not get through at all. This problem is further compounded when we realize that the severity of the hearing loss, the background noise, the acoustics of a room, fatigue, and the absence of appropriate assistive devices can change not only how hearing-impaired people hear sounds, but what sounds they hear on any given day.

What can you do to improve this situation? Probably more than you think. If your hearing loss at this point is relatively slight, chances are you are missing such small pieces of conversation that you can still get the topic and guess your way through the rest. But if your hearing has deteriorated or if you have already reached the point where one-third to one-half of what you hear in conversation sounds like a computer talking to a blue jay, then you might consider redefining sound. In other words, you may wish to begin teaching yourself how to transform the static, squawks, and whirs, or the mushy and indistinct noises you now hear into meaningful sound.

Can this be done? Yes. Can it be done in two months and twelve easy lessons? No, because a hearing loss is often not stable; what you can understand today may become gibberish tomorrow. By the same token, hearing aids are getting better and better, and what are blips and squeals today just might become words next year. The point is, until a better answer is found for your particular problem, you will need to work at exploring what you can hear, what is distorted, and what you cannot hear. Since this may become a lifelong task, let me explain how we learn and how it applies to hearing-impaired people.

Finding the Meaning in Sound Signals

Imagine that you are a baby and you have just started to hear for the first time. You hear lots of noises, but because you cannot identify them you do not know what they mean. Every sound is a surprise, every noise is different, for you do not yet know the categories of sounds (Vygotsky, 1962). As we grow, we learn to classify the sounds we hear. For example, a starling does not sound like a jay, but you and I would know them both as birds. A metal pan being dropped on a linoleum floor sounds similar to a pair of pliers being dropped, and we classify these as unbreakable things being dropped on a hard floor (Britton, 1970). If you do not know what sounds are, then they are just noises. You know that something made a noise, but you have no way of classifying that noise. Since no two noises are absolutely identical, a baby hears thousands of unique noises (Piaget, 1976).

This is very confusing in several ways. First of all, if you have a hearing loss you, like the baby, cannot identify noise as something meaningful, it startles you. You may even jump and look around, trying to identify the cause of the noise. You are not trying to remember the noise or analyze it, you are trying to identify it (Britton, 1970). You want to know if the noise indicates danger or indicates you need to do something, such as answer the door or pick up the pieces of the vase the cat knocked off the bookshelf. When we are startled, we concentrate on identifying what caused the noise rather than the noise itself. This is because of the relationship between the brain and the mind and their respective functions.

The ear picks up sound waves and transports them along the auditory nerve so the brain can understand the signal. The brain recognizes the signal for noise, and the mind analyzes the signal and tries to identify it. When the sound is not immediately recognized by the mind, the mind flashes a warning signal. The mind does not know what the sound is, and until the sound is identified, the cause of the sound is potentially life threatening (Britton, 1970; Costello, 1982). This is an example of how the brain and the mind work together to keep us safe from the dangers of the world. If a sound cannot be identified, the mind and brain want us to be alert in case we have to do something to escape danger. That slight rush you feel after being startled is from the adrenaline that the brain has ordered your body to release into your system to give you top muscle performance. Your heartbeat quickens and you take a quick deep breath, which pumps oxygen into your system so you can react to the danger, whatever it is.

While all this is going on, you are using all your senses—sight, smell, touch, and hearing—to try to identify the sound. Because all this happens, we sometimes have a hard time remembering exactly what the noise sounded like. If we identify the sound (for example, a car backfiring) the first time, then it becomes more likely we will identify the sound the second time. After several repetitions of the incident, we can reach the point at which we are no longer badly startled (even though we may be startled at first) when we hear a car backfire as we are walking along a busy street.

Now imagine this process in a person who wears hearing aids that distort some noises by making them louder and completely unrecognizable. A spoon falling and bouncing off a linoleum floor could sound like lightning striking the chimney. A door slamming in the wind could sound like a truck hitting the side of the house. Common, everyday sounds that never used to bother that person become things that go bump in the night, noises that startle. And if a person is startled enough times and cannot identify the noises, he or she can become fearful, anxious, or on edge at the least noise (Costello, 1982; Shaughnessy, 1977).

Loud noises are not the only sounds that can startle. After all, we do not memorize every sound we've ever heard. We identify classes of sounds, sounds that have similar causes, sounds that share relationships (Piaget, 1976). This identification process begins when we are babies. For example, a baby tries to figure out what sound its mother makes. The baby can recognize its mother's voice long before it knows what she is saying. The baby does not have to know all the possible sounds a mommy can make, just that this sort of sound is Mommy (Britton, 1970).

The baby listens for the differences between sounds. If the differences are not too great, the baby will start to lump the individual sounds into sound groups. This kind of fine discrimination takes a long time to learn. When we learn to discriminate, the first thing we try to determine is what is different. We usually look for gross differences, like the difference between a bell ringing and a jet taking off. One sound is rhythmic, the other steady and building. One sound is pleasant, the other overwhelming (Vygotsky, 1962).

Problems arise if the sounds are not grossly different. If the sounds are similar (say, as a bird squawking and a door squeaking), and we cannot immediately identify the class of the sounds, then by the time we figure out what that sound was, we have forgotten what it sounded like. This is because our mind and brain were concentrating on identification, not on remembering (Costello, 1981–1984; Howards, 1980).

Corrupted Signals

As the distortions of the sounds perceived become greater, the ability to identify changes in these sounds decreases. The brain continues to pick up the sounds even though they are very much changed from the sounds the mind once knew. The problem is that the mind has a harder and harder time identifying the differences and similarities between these sounds. If the mind does not identify sound, the sound itself is forgotten as the mind and brain try desperately to identify it. In addition to not being able to identify the sound, the mind will not be able to remember it the next time.

As this happens over and over again, the mind starts to get very confused. The brain continues to relay the signals, but the mind just cannot interpret them. It is as if the mind says to itself, "Well, I just can't get it. I know it was a sound because I see someone talking to me. And I know that the sound is supposed to be language because I'm interpreting all the other messages that the brain is giving me. But that particular sound is unidentifiable as a language sound. And so is that one. Now, that sounded like *toad-*

stool, but because I didn't get the two sounds that came before it, can that possibly be right?"

Gradually this listener's mind becomes more and more doubtful of its ability to identify the fine differences between sounds, such as *t* and *s* (Smith, 1978; Shaughnessy, 1977). So, the mind starts to look for big differences, and the problem then becomes that in any given language, there aren't any. But that does not stop the mind from looking for them. By ignoring the small differences between the sounds, the mind literally "does not hear them." The brain picks them up, but the mind ignores them, so they are lost at almost the same instant they are perceived. The listener identifies less and less, confusing the mind more and more, and sound discrimination becomes worse and worse (Smith, 1978; Shaughnessy, 1977).

In trying to identify everything, the mind has created a situation that makes it difficult for it to identify anything (Howards, 1980; Shaughnessy, 1977). The mind stops looking for the tiny differences, such as those between *carpet* and *carport,* and looks instead for the big differences, such as identifying whether someone is talking or coughing.

Straightening Out the Signals

If you are struggling to identify the sounds that your hearing aid and/or hearing loss have distorted, you need to reteach yourself to hear differences. This is not as straightforward as it sounds. The brain and mind work hard to identify sounds, a process that involves a series of critical steps that occur in rapid succession without our being aware of them. The first thing you must do is *not* try to identify sounds. It does not matter what the sounds are; what matters is what the sounds are like (Vygotsky, 1962).

This advice runs contrary to the methods taught in many of the speech discrimination programs designed for hard of hearing people. These programs tend to focus on sound identification, but that is the *last* step of the mental process of sound discrimination, not the first! Our goal is to work with the brain and the mind, as much as we are able, to learn the way they learn, in the order that they learn it.

We will start by explaining what the brain and mind do when they try to make sense of noise. All sound is recognized as noise at first because noise is sound without meaning. The brain and mind have learned that, and have not forgotten it. The incoming sound signal travels from the hearing aids and/or ears along pathways of nerves to the brain, where it is noticed by the mind. Next, the brain and the mind start working together to discover why that noise is different from all the other sounds and noises they are dealing with at this particular second.

In order to discriminate between sounds, we need to perceive their differences. People with a hearing loss must relearn the differences in sound. They need to start to listen for the shape of sound. Just like a baby, they need to investigate the sound of sound (Britton, 1970).

You encounter sounds every day that may be distorted, such as a spoon dropping or a doorbell ringing. So drop a spoon on your kitchen floor and listen! Listen for the sound and try to identify its qualities: Is it hard or soft? High or low? Sharp or smooth? Big or small? Was it a single, cohesive sound, or did it have several parts to it?

The next time you climb into your car and start the engine, listen. If you see a dog barking, listen. As you become better at noticing sound as sound, you will become better at both understanding and identifying what you hear and do not hear. You will also remember sounds in their new shapes.

If you hear a sound you don't recognize, don't worry. Just listen, look around, and identify the source, if you can. If you cannot identify the source and there are people near you (whom you don't mind asking), ask them what the noise was. You will make the most progress at recognizing sounds if you already know what or where the noise is coming from before you listen. In these situations you do not have to worry about identifying the sound, so you can concentrate more fully on the sound itself.

You do a hundred things every day that create sound. Think of just the first half-hour of your day. That is an almost complete lesson in the sounds water can make! Have you ever stopped to listen to the sound that a flushing toilet makes? First it goes *hur-rummm* as the first water is released. Then it goes *rummsh-rummsh-rummsh-rummsh* as the water goes around and around. Then it goes *blump . . . . blump . . . blump . . blump . blump-blump-blump* as the last of the water bubbles away. Finally, it goes *shshshshshshshshshshshshsh* as the water is pushed back in. The bathroom is a veritable treasure-trove of sound, from the toilet, the shower, the faucet, and the water draining out of the tub after a bath.

Why should you listen to water in the bathroom? Because you are trying to relearn a class of sounds—the sounds that water makes. These waterlike sounds are all around us—sprinklers, rain in gutters, rivers and streams, someone washing a car. If you can identify the sound class water, then you stand a much better chance of recognizing many different environmental sounds.

Knowing the sound class is a bit like knowing the topic. If you know the topic, then you can predict the words. If you know the kinds of sounds water can make, then you are much more likely to identify the water sound you hear in a particular setting.

Another benefit of paying attention to sounds is that you will be helping your mind learn to pay attention to sound. And if you are relaxed, and best of all, having some fun with the whole thing, your mind will pay attention and learn. This is an important point. Testing, as I am sure you realize, is not fun. Even testing yourself (I'm going to sit here with my eyes closed and see if I can identify the next sound) is not really fun. The reason is that even if no one is around to notice whether or not you managed to name the noise, you will know that you either succeeded or failed. *Test* implies success or failure, and failure is not very comfortable. So try not to test yourself (Costello, 1981–1984).

Learning happens best in an atmosphere of relaxation, and if possible, of fun or happiness. We tend not to learn very much if we are upset, nervous, or anxious, or afraid of failure (Costello, 1981–1984; Robinson, 1981–1983).

As you rediscover and redefine sound, you will begin to be more aware of the sounds that are around us all the time, and you will be better able to discriminate between them. Noticing sounds is very important. It will let you know quickly when background noises begin to drown out an important conversation. It will help you be more comfortable with, and at the same time more aware of, your surroundings. And maybe, just maybe, it will extend the time you can comfortably wear your hearing aids before you become anxious or fatigued.

Encouraging Signal Recognition

Our brains and minds are really wonderful. If we work with them in ways they recognize, they will do awe-inspiring things for us. One of the most complex things they do for us is allow us to

understand and use language. Since, as adults, we already understand and use language, it is not necessary for us to relearn the
whole process. All we need to do is get the mind started on the
right track and keep it there, and it will move along all by itself. We
do not need to teach the mind how to recognize differences, we
just give it the room to do so by noticing the textures of sound, by
being relaxed and in good humor, and by working with it (keeping
the topic and predicting) instead of against it (testing) (Vygotsky,
1962; Britton, 1970).

Your brain and mind together have been recognizing differences and similarities for years now. Because of your hearing loss,
you need to encourage them to relearn sound. You can get them
on the right track by noticing how sounds are different and how
different sounds can sometimes be inside of one sound. Labeling
sounds (*scratchy, thumping, smooth*), helps the mind remember the
differences. Then, the mind becomes better and better at noticing
the sounds until it can distinguish finer and finer differences.
Once the mind notices the differences in sounds, it begins to
notice the similarities between sounds. When you reach this point,
your mind is able to classify sounds by grouping like sounds together into categories. This, then, is the goal—to be able to recognize a sound class (Vygotsky, 1962). It will take time and hard,
creative work, but you can reach that goal if you encourage the
mind's exploration in an atmosphere of relaxation.

Nine

Working Within and Beyond the Limitations

We can think of the mind as an overseer, a quick acting decision maker. It looks at the signals the brain receives and makes a number of judgments about them. Then, it draws on memory to try to identify those signals. When the mind does identify a signal, that signal becomes meaningful to us. We recognize it, and as in the case of the word *cat*, associate a whole string of thoughts with that meaningful signal (Vygotsky, 1962; Costello, 1982).

Let me give you an example of this process at work. As I sat at my computer, writing to you about the brain and the mind, my ears picked up a signal. It was a faint scratchy sound, not squeaky, but not soft, either. The signal came from my right, but not from the bedroom. Therefore, it must have been a sound in the entry way or the living room. My ears sent this information to my brain in an instant, my brain transformed the signal into something my mind could recognize, my mind identified the sound as something familiar to me, and in less than a second, I knew my cat was scratching at the front door to be let in. This is how meaning is created—signal to brain, to mind, to identification, to meaning, all in the blink of an eye! But that's not the end of it.

My next thoughts were that (1) I had to get up and let the cat in, (2) I had to finish typing this thought, (3) I should forget the cat; she would only want to go right back out again, (4) Wow! This was a perfect and real example of what I was writing about!

This is what happens when everything is working just the way it is supposed to, but we know very well that our senses and the brain and the mind do not always get it right. In chapter 8 we looked at the signal, the brain, and the mind, and their relationship. In this chapter we are going to add another piece of the puzzle—memory.

Memory is the accumulation of thoughts. It is like a giant library card catalogue, where everything is referenced and cross-referenced so that one thought leads to another and another and another. Our memories are our own private repositories, our storehouses for everything we have seen, smelled, or heard, everything we have experienced that touched us in a meaningful way, including our dreams. But until information gets into memory, it is of no use to us (Campbell, 1982; Piaget, 1978).

The more you know about the nature of memory—how it works and what its limitations are—the better you will understand your reactions to communication. You also will gain insight into why you might feel tired or irritable when you try to keep up with a conversation, and why you can hear better on some days, or even at certain times of the day, than others.

We are used to thinking of memory as one entity, but it is really composed of different parts. Short-term memory is one part. It is where signals are first put together to make meaning. Long-term memory is the storage place for everything that short-term memory understands and passes on.

To understand how short- and long-term memory work together, let's look at an example. Short-term memory needs input in order to start working. Since reading is input, we'll use a written sentence as our example: Two black horses cantered through the meadow.

As your eyes move across the message, short-term memory works with the brain and mind to try to create meaning. It does this by working in chunks (Smith, 1978). The first chunk might be "two black horses," and because you can create meaning from that, short-term memory switches it through to long-term memory. Then, the whole process starts again on the next chunk, which may be "cantered through the meadow." Again, meaning is recognized, so this chunk is passed through. The difference between fast and not-so-fast readers is that fast readers would see the whole input sentence as one chunk, while slower readers would break it up into several chunks (Smith, 1971; Howards, 1980).

This process only works if meaning can be created in short-term memory. If, for some reason, meaning cannot be created, then the whole process comes to a screeching halt. Let me show you.

I am going to present two chunks, each with the identical number of letters. What I want you to do is read each set once, just as you are reading this sentence. Read at normal speed and read the chunks only once. Then slap your hand over the chunks to cover up the letters and see if you can remember any part of the chunks. Ready? Okay, give it a try.

The maple trees are starting to turn color
Rno gesee ortnr elt luiaepto th racr tmats

Do you remember what was in the first chunk? Do you remember what it was about? Do you think you remember it word for word? How about the second chunk? Do you remember how many parts there were to the chunk? Do you remember any of the words? Odds are, you remembered a great deal more about the first chunk than the second. In fact, you may even be able to completely reproduce the first chunk in your own handwriting. How about the second? If you cannot remember a thing about the second, congratulations: you are normal. If you do remember a bit of it, then pat yourself on the back, for you are a careful reader with a wonderful memory. Now go ahead and uncover the chunks.

The two chunks had the identical number of parts, the identical number of letters, and they even had identical letters. The difference was that the first chunk had those letters arranged in such a way that, if you know how to read English, they are potentially meaningful. But the second chunk was arranged so it could not be meaningful (Jacobs and Rosenbaum, 1971; Howards, 1980).

Meaningful signals, signals that are recognized by the mind as creating a picture or a thought, are transferred from short-term to long-term memory. Gibberish is rarely, if ever, transferred. Usually, it is rejected, dumped out of short-term memory, and forgotten (Smith, 1978; Costello, 1982). This is so important I am going to repeat it. Only meaningful information gets transferred from short- to long-term memory.

Now let's look at how memory works and why understanding the limitations of memory is so very important to hearing-impaired people.

Long-Term Memory

When meaning is created in short-term memory, that meaning is shifted from short-term memory to long-term memory. When we think of memory, we most often think of long-term memory. Long-term memory stores all of the meaningful bits and pieces that we receive from short-term memory, and then organizes them so we have a chance of finding them again. It organizes the information according to what is important to us (Howards, 1980; Chomsky, 1960).

No two people organize their memories just the same way because each of us is different, and what is important to one person might be unimportant to another. The length of time a piece of information remains accessible to each of us is dependent on how important that information is to each individual person (Paulk, 1984). For example, I am sure I saw on the evening news what the price of gold was on today's market; I remember seeing the arrows and numbers on the stock market report, yet I do not remember what that price was. However, a broker who buys and sells precious metals would remember. It is important to the broker and not particularly important to me.

In a sense, all minds create meaning equally, but we all store it in our own individual ways, according to how we see the world around us and what is important to each of us as individuals.

Short-Term Memory

Short-term memory has severe limitations, and these limitations can have an especially strong impact on hearing-impaired people. First of all, short-term memory has a small capacity. It can hold only about seven items. Those items can be words, letters, numbers, or bits of meaning, but seven is about the limit. Second, short-term memory can only hold those few items for a couple of seconds. If it cannot create meaning in one or two seconds, then it dumps the items to get ready for the next items (Smith, 1978; Howards, 1971).

Most of the time short-term memory is so good at making meaning that we don't notice it working at all. It takes its items or chunks, makes meaning, then transfers the meaning to long-term memory, all so smoothly we don't even realize we have more than one kind of memory.

If we want to remember something that is not meaningful, then we have to memorize it by repeating it time and time again (Smith, 1978). Here is an example: Suppose you are in a phone booth. You need to make a call, but you don't have the number. You also don't have a pencil or paper, and the phone book is missing. You call directory assistance, and the operator gives you the number. You need to remember that number just long enough to place the call, so while you fish another quarter out of your pocket, you repeat the number to yourself, over and over again. Since phone numbers are not meaningful (do not create pictures in our minds), we have to remember them by rote. We hold the number sequence in short-term memory by repeating it faster than short-term memory can dump it out. And if our attention is distracted in any way, ooops! There goes the phone number.

What would happen if a fire engine were to go screaming past your phone booth, sirens blaring, just as you deposited the quarter to make the call? Chances are you would be startled, short-term memory would wipe itself clean, take in the information about the fire truck, send all relevant data concerning the fire truck to your mind for identification and evaluation, and then pay attention to the truck long enough for the mind to calculate whether or not you were in danger from this noisy "beast." By then, you have forgotten the phone number!

Short-term memory is rather like a chalkboard that our senses are continually writing on. In order to make enough room for all of the information, it works very quickly and wipes itself clean every few seconds to be ready for the next piece of meaningful information. This happens automatically and continuously. In order to hold information in short-term memory, you must constantly repeat the information (a phone number, an address, a shopping list) to yourself; in other words, keep putting it back up on the self-erasing chalkboard. If your attention wanders from this task, the information is lost.

When information is lost because it is not understood in the brief amount of time short-term memory allows for understanding, the mind can get upset or confused. Remember, the mind's job is to use meaning to make sense of the world. That is what it wants to do, and that is what you want it to do. If information is lost just once in a while, it is no big deal. Usually additional input (the next sentence, for example) will clear up what was missed. But if two chunks in a row are missed, then a problem develops. The listener can become anxious and will focus even more attention on what is being said. This is a deadly loop.

The Deadly Loop

The whole process from signal to short-term memory to recognition to long-term memory works best if the listener is relaxed and receptive. The more nervous the listener, the more restricted the process.

All of us have been in situations where we felt we just could not stuff one more bit of information into our minds. When we work hard to keep up with something for a long time, we tire physically and mentally. If we try to keep going—to the next lecture, the next meeting, the next project—we can become so fatigued that short-term memory simply refuses to keep up. It stops shifting information to long-term memory and, as a result, our intellect suffers. The most obvious things just do not seem to register.

When I try to cook after a long and tiring day, a dish that normally takes me half an hour to prepare can take me as much as an hour. I cannot remember where a certain pot is, cannot remember if I have already added the oregano, and have a tendency to salt things twice. Granted, those are little things, but they do not help my disposition or my digestion.

The bottom line is that when we tire, we do not make meaning as well as when we are fresh. The complex operations of making meaning and getting that meaning to long-term memory become harder and harder as we become more fatigued (Howards, 1980; Costello, 1981–1984).

This problem is compounded for people who are hearing-impaired. They want so badly to make sense out of what they hear that they send the sounds through short-term memory again and again. This attempt to make meaning requires concentrating all efforts on remembering, reviewing, and making sense. And the heartbreaking part of all this is that if someone cannot make meaning out of the chunk, short-term memory will dump the sounds out of memory, and the person will not recall those little bits and pieces that might have helped make the next chunk heard meaningful. It is all gone (Smith, 1978).

Without a base of meaning from the first chunk of sound, it becomes less and less likely that a hearing-impaired person will understand the second, third, or fourth chunk of sound. That is why it is so important to have the topic in mind. It provides clues so the listener can predict and better understand the next chunk.

Because short-term memory has size and time limitations, the mind does not have time to do much more than one task. But when we miss the first chunk of meaning, we tend to concentrate more energy on listening. In essence, we are forcing the mind to listen at the same time that short-term memory is trying to create meaning from sounds that are meaningless. As a result, we become more and more distressed, and we tend to concentrate on smaller and smaller chunks of signal. It is as if we were saying to ourselves, "Well, I couldn't understand that six-item chunk, so I'll only include three or four items in the next chunk." The problem with this approach is that our language often takes five, six, or seven chunks (or words) to create meaning (Smith, 1978).

As an example, let's take a look at a pair of words to see if you can guess their meaning—was going. Well? Yes, you can read the words, but what do they mean? Do these two words carry enough meaning for you to make a mental picture? Is there meaning that you can identify with? Remember, you only had two or three seconds to find that meaning. But what if you were a bit more relaxed and got four words in one chunk: was going to the?

That is not much better. You can begin to see that one of the problems associated with listening for every word means you are listening for a lot of structural words that potentially do not have much to do with the message. (We talked about this in chapter 7.) Suppose, though, that you are really relaxed and as receptive as you can be. You pick up all the words it is possible for you to get in one chunk, so that you hear all at once: was going to the dentist fun?

Now that was a message! It has everything you need to create meaning. You have a question that the speaker wants you to respond to, and you understood it in one chunk. You did not have to put meaningless sounds on hold while you waited for the next chunk to complete the meaning.

Our minds and memories are truly wonderful, and they will work very hard for us if we give them a chance. They will even help us ignore unimportant words, such as *the,* so we can get more words in each chunk of short-term memory, making it more possible for us to create meaning. This is as true for people with normal hearing as it is for people with a hearing loss. But the more trouble a person has understanding speech, the more necessary it becomes to not listen too hard for every little sound.

Getting distressed and listening to every sound fills up the capacity of short-term memory too quickly with bits of language that mean little by themselves. That makes it less likely that a hearing-impaired listener will create meaning, which will make the listener more anxious, which causes her to focus harder on even smaller bits, which makes it less likely she will create meaning (Howards, 1980; Smith, 1978). The longer this continues, the more stressful communication becomes. This is the deadly loop.

This whole problem is made even worse by trying to hold sounds in short-term memory by repeating them in the hopes of identifying them the second or third time around. Concentrating so hard that the sounds are sent through short-term memory again and again not only causes fatigue but also results in the loss of all the other things being said in the meantime. A person who is concentrating on what was already said can no longer use prediction because he is not listening for what could come next.

The sheer work that hearing-impaired people have to put forth to understand conversation in any circumstance is tremendous. They are straining their minds every second of every conversation, doing three or five or ten times more work than a person with normal hearing would have to do. Add to this already tense situation the problems created when a person focuses too hard on all the little sounds, and you have the potential for major problems. The hearing-impaired person struggles harder and harder to create meaning, looking at smaller and smaller chunks in the hopes of understanding each word. But as the chunks contain less and less information, they are more likely to be dumped from short-term memory, never getting the chance to transfer to long-term memory. The frustration levels rise, the listener comprehends less, and focuses more and more on smaller and smaller pieces of information (Howards, 1980; Shaughnessy, 1977). This deadly loop can also create the physical symptoms of stress.

Stopping the Deadly Loop

Our minds work to keep us safe. When we start to get overloaded, our minds react by telling us to back off and by shutting down. Some people become forgetful, others get nervous and tired. The best thing to do in this situation is to stop what you are doing. Take off your hearing aids and relax for ten minutes. Go do something that does not require you to identify sounds—read a book, do some gardening, write a letter, take a nap, clean the house, walk around the block or down to the brook, or go to a store and browse. If you do not stop what you are doing, the reaction to overloading will just keep getting worse and worse (Costello, 1982).

The amount of time you can spend concentrating on conversation will depend upon many factors—how much your hearing impairment interferes with understanding speech, whether or not you had a good night's sleep, whether or not the speaker is careful and considerate, how prepared you are for the conversation, and how familiar or comfortable you are with the speaker's speech patterns and/or the topic. Even if you are rested, the speaker is careful, the acoustics are good, and you know the topic, two or three dumps by short-term memory can start the anxiety level climbing.

The key is to be relaxed and open to communication. The more relaxed and receptive you are, the more work your mind can do for you, the more associations it can make with what it has to work with in short-term memory, and the more items short-term memory can hold for you. Both of these factors will greatly increase your chances of making meaning (Campbell, 1982; Smith, 1971).

What it all comes down to is that you have to listen to yourself. You have to judge when you can and when you cannot concentrate. At the end of a long and trying day you may need to say, "I'm so tired, I'm just not able to follow any more conversations. I don't have any energy left." You may need to learn ways of saving the things you want to talk about with friends or family or business colleagues for when you feel fresh. You may need to be careful about making appointments; for example, do not schedule more than one appointment in any given day; leave fifteen minutes, half an hour, or an hour in between appointments; or make important or special meetings in the morning or afternoon only.

You may find that some simple relaxation techniques (deep breathing, thinking of a special place, or light meditation) can significantly lengthen the amount of time you can spend listening in "one go." If your work requires you to sit through long (half-hour or more) meetings, or if you just want to be able to keep up with the family for a whole evening, I strongly urge you to look into relaxation techniques. The American Tinnitus Association has an excellent booklet on basic relaxation techniques, and many health care organizations and community colleges give workshops to help people reduce stress.

The fatigue you experience after talking to someone is real. It is a result of pushing yourself to a high level of mental concentration over a period of time in potentially frustrating situations (Goldberger and Bresnitz, 1982). The amount of time you can concentrate this hard and not begin to feel stress will vary from day to day, and even from hour to hour. This is the major reason why on some days you can hear very well and on other days nothing makes sense. It is also why, with everything else equal, what you clearly can understand in the morning you may not be able to understand at night.

I cannot stress strongly enough that the fatigue a hard of hearing person experiences when trying to follow spoken communication is a genuine, honest feeling. Imagine taking three, two-hour college final exams in one day. Can you imagine how numb you would be? This is the kind of exhaustion that the hearing-impaired person can be feeling at the end of any reasonably busy day. By this time, a hearing-impaired person may be "all used up," so exhausted from making meaning all day long that he or she just cannot do it any more. Unfortunately, this is the time many people set aside for family communication.

The problem of not being able to understand or track conversation is not, however, limited to fatigue or stress. Often, a physical reaction or allergy to a food or a noisy or acoustically poor environment can cause a hearing-impaired person to lose even more hearing. A common head cold can interfere to the point that the slender hold a person had on communication is lost altogether.

The key to communication is understanding. If hard of hearing people can better understand why they tire quickly and why they cannot hear very well in a particular situation, then they can communicate that to the people around them. This takes some thought and research on their part. They must understand and define their needs, and they can only do that by paying attention to themselves and those around them.

Once a hearing-impaired person has identified his or her personal levels of fatigue, he or she will know when to take a break from listening and trying to interpret spoken communication. The next step is to work on reducing the stress inherent in daily, face-to-face communication. Many excellent pamphlets, books, and classes are available on this topic. The best advice we can offer you is to make use of them.

In our experience, hearing-impaired people who can identify and head off stress quickly markedly increase the amount of time they can effectively communicate. In essence, they stop the deadly loop at its onset, never letting it fully develop to its potentially exhausting conclusion.

Ten

Language, Power, and Politeness

In our society, quick witted people are often perceived as able to get things done. Corporate America rewards people who can think on their feet; in other words, understand and execute directives with a minimum of information (input) and at maximum speed. Teachers grow impatient with the students who take a moment or two before answering questions (What's the matter; didn't he understand the question? Didn't she study? Is he stupid, a little slow?). We wonder about quiet people (What's the matter; doesn't she care about this?). We persecute shy people (Come on, speak up. Don't you have anything to say for yourself?). Given the fact that we often judge people not only by what they say, but by how they respond to what we say, the hearing-impaired person who has trouble with spoken communication can legitimately feel at a disadvantage.

Missing the words is more than not understanding a sentence. It strikes at the very core of our self-esteem. "I don't understand" is equated with "I'm not smart." Is it any wonder that hearing-impaired people are reluctant to say, "I don't understand"? Is it any wonder that many of them begin to lose confidence? Remember how you felt when you got your English composition papers back and they were covered with comments written in red pen, comments like *awkward, run-on sentence, split infinitive, fragment,* and *example?* Well, missing words in conversation is worse. The people you speak to have the red pen; they can judge you and mark you down for errors you did not know you made, with a finality you cannot fight.

In this chapter I am going to present an overview of language to give you an insight into the components of spoken language. I will explain how language is used to pass information from one person to another, to create and define social conventions such as politeness, and to create and define each person's place in relationship to others. Based on this information, I will then explain how a hearing loss results in much more than missing a word or two.

Keep in mind that this is just a quick introduction to the study of spoken language, based on the work of a few select researchers. There is an enormous amount of information written about language, so I have decided to focus only on those aspects that I believe directly concern a person who has a hearing loss.

The bibliography at the end of this book lists sources that provide a more detailed and complete understanding of the uses to which we put language and how those uses define and redefine each of us according to the communication situation in which we find ourselves. For those who want to explore this topic further, these sources can give great insights into our use of language and how it shapes us.

The Three Levels of Spoken Communication

In face-to-face, spoken communication, language simultaneously operates on at least three levels. The first level has such names as semantics, social semiotics, grammatical conventions (which include transformational as well as other grammars), linguistics, and verbal linguistics. The second level is called paralinguistics, vocal communication, nonlinguistic elements, and metalinguistics, among other things. The third level is most often referred to as either kinesics or nonvocal communication.

All these terms are used not because professionals can't agree, but because language is so complex. The concept we glibly call *meaning* is also complex and highly individual. No two people define words exactly the same way or want to convey the exact same meaning. So, any truth pertaining to language will by nature tend to be a generalization that is bound by generalizations (Lyons, 1977).

In terms of generalizations, a great deal of information is available that can illuminate what language is and how we use it (including how it can be used to help or to hurt us). For the purposes of this chapter, I am going to choose among the names and definitions of each of the three levels and present my own generalization.

Level One: The Words and Structures

When most people think of language, they think of words and structures. We choose the words to convey the meaning we want to get across. The structures are the arrangements of those words into sentences (or phrases or clauses).

The Words

English is rich in words. In fact, many words can be used to describe the same thing. The study of the words we choose to use is *semantics.* The reason we choose one word over another may be as simple as choosing the easiest word for us or the first word we happen to think of that fits the situation, but often we make the choice based on a variety of factors.

For example, let's look at the word *cat.* If we were being very proper, or sarcastic, we could say *domestic feline. Kitty* is an affectionate term, as is *kitty-cat,* either of which we might choose out of fondness or because we are talking to a very young child. I could use any of those words to describe my cat, since they are all perfectly good words.

My husband David and I have a cat. Her name is Crystal, but we also call her a number of other things, such as *Chris, fur-face, fleabag,* and *scuz-ball.* These are all terms of affection. Our word choice depends on where we are, how we are talking about her, what instigated the conversation about her (describing her to someone else or talking directly to her after she has done something particularly dumb or amusing), and who else (besides the cat) is in on the conversation. Given all these variables (and many more) I would choose the name (or noun) not only to describe the cat as the subject of the conversation, but to give further information concerning how I feel about her at that particular moment (Lyons, 1977).

The Structures

Just as we can choose different words, we can put those words into different structures. The study of language structure is *syntax,* or grammar. We are going to look at a specific kind of grammar—transformational grammar—to get an understanding of the structure of language and how the structures we choose help us to create different meanings (Chomsky, 1968).

Before we begin, I would like to introduce a linguistic term that will be useful to our discussion. The term is *utterance,* and it refers to everything a person says during one turn of talking (Searle, 1972).

For example, suppose Fred and Larry are having a conversation. In this conversation, they will take turns talking. First Fred will say something, then Larry will say something. Fred may say just one word, like "Hello!" Then Larry might reply, "Hi. Nice day, isn't it?" Fred's one word was his turn, so it is an utterance. Larry's turn, or reply, even though it included five words, is also an utterance (Goody, 1978).

The term *utterance* is more appropriate for our discussion because we do not always speak in sentences, and sometimes we say a lot more than just one sentence. An utterance can be a sound (uh-huh), a word, or forty sentences. The utterance is defined by one person taking a turn in a conversation, not by the number of words spoken.

The dialogue that follows shows how structures modify or change the meaning of our messages.

> *Participants:* Fred and Larry have been co-workers for about three years, but are not friends outside the office. They are managers of equal standing, each in different areas. Fred is in marketing and Larry is in finance.
>
> *Setting:* Larry's office, where Fred and Larry are having a cup of coffee.
>
> *Topic:* A new junior manager has just been hired. This is of interest to both Fred and Larry because the new junior manager will probably be training under one or both of them.

(1) *Fred:* "Have you heard that a new junior manager's been hired?"
(2) *Larry:* "Yes, and Janice, whose opinion I respect, says she's a good find for the company."
(3) *Fred:* "Oh, she's a woman? I hadn't heard that."
(4) *Larry:* "Yes. From what I hear, she's a graduate from Stanford in Marketing and Management."

Now let's examine what could be going on in this conversation, one utterance at a time.

(1) Fred: "Have you heard that a new junior manager's been hired?"—Several different structures could be used here that would still retain all the words. Fred could have said, "Have you heard? A new junior manager's been hired." This statement is much stronger than the one that Fred used partly because it is a statement rather than a question—"A new junior manager's been hired," rather than, "Have you heard that a new junior manager's been hired?" Making the whole utterance a question, as Fred did, allows Fred to give information about the utterance beyond the words he spoke (Soames and Perlmutter, 1979).

First, Fred could have been trying to deliver the information politely and kindly. Saying the whole utterance as a question makes it seem less like common knowledge and more like the latest news that not everyone would be expected to know. It gives Larry a way to say, "No, I didn't know," and not sound uninformed or behind the times (Goody, 1978).

Second, by phrasing the utterance as a question, Fred was making it clear that he expected a response from Larry, and he gave Larry the room to respond. It is often more difficult to respond to a statement. If Fred said, "Did you hear? A new junior manager's been hired," Larry should respond to "Did you hear?" and that needs only a yes or no answer. By using the statement form, Fred would not be inviting Larry to take part in a pleasant conversation. In fact, he would be limiting Larry's role in the conversation (Goody, 1978). Fred would more likely be using the statement to find out if Larry knew about the new manager. He could even be showing off superior knowledge.

(2) Larry: "Yes, and Janice, whose opinion I respect, says she's a good find for the company."—This was Larry's response to Fred's question. Let's take a look at the structure of this sentence. First of all, we have four different remarks. The first one is the response to the question that Fred posed, which is yes. The second is "Janice says," identifying the source of the information about to be given. The third is "she's a good find for the company," which gives information about the topic. The fourth is "I respect Janice's opinion," which gives the speaker's opinion of the source of the information (Bennett, 1976; Goody, 1978).

The part of the utterance with the most interesting structures is Janice, whose opinion I respect, says. . . ." The clause—whose opinion I respect—is called a *transformed sentence*. The original sentence before the transformation was "I respect her opinion." In order to put this inside another sentence, as Larry did, it must be transformed into an adjective clause. English has specific rules for creating an adjective clause, rules that we use every day and don't even think about (see Bornstein, 1972, and Robinson, 1983 for more information). After Larry transformed the sentence into the clause, he inserted (or embedded) the clause into another sentence.

Now, why did Larry do that? Why didn't he just say "Yes, and Janice says she's a good find for the company. I respect Janice's opinion." It would seem that the utterance is easier to say this way instead of going through the process of transformating and embedding. So there should be a reason why Larry would take the trouble to do this, and there is.

In the original utterance, Larry was basically saying that he respected the source of his information (Janice). It is as if Larry is confirming what he and Fred both know—Janice is reliable and trustworthy (Lyons, 1977; Soames and Perlmutter, 1979).

If Larry had chosen to say at the end of his utterance, "I respect Janice's opinion," rather than transform and embed the statement, then he would have been giving a different signal. He would have been putting emphasis on the fact that he respects Janice's opinion. In other words, Larry might have been conveying the message that while he felt that Janice was trustworthy, he was not sure that Fred would know it or agree with him. He would be asserting his opinion of the source, rather than trying to confirm mutual agreement of the source. By asserting his opinion, Larry could be challenging Fred verbally with an "I believe this, and you'd better too if you know what's good for you" kind of attitude (Goody, 1978; Elgin, 1980).

In summary, "I respect Janice's opinion" is much more assertive and potentially hostile. It almost begs for Fred to respond, either by agreeing and confirming Larry's knowledge/belief or by disagreeing and thereby, in effect, telling Larry that his belief in Janice's trustworthiness is wrong (and if Fred did that, he could also be calling Larry a bad judge of character).

By using the transformation and embedding the assertion, Larry makes Janice's trustworthiness more of a shared opinion, as though he were mentioning something they were both aware of. Also, by embedding it, Larry is letting Fred off the hook. If Fred does not agree, he can simply keep silent. We do not have to respond to embedded statements; they are very easy to ignore. And while we often do not have to respond to statements, either, some statements (especially ones like this) are ploys for approval or power. By not responding to them, we might feel we have been put in our place or made to feel inferior (Bennett, 1976; Elgin, 1980).

(3) Fred: "Oh, she's a woman? I hadn't heard that."—By now, you have probably gotten the idea that a question is potentially much more polite than a statement. And so it is. A natural alternative to the way Fred structured his utterance is "I hadn't heard that she's a woman." Fred could have said the alternative in a very straightforward manner (with no snide or angry overtones), and it probably would have come out sounding pretty much the same as the original. But the alternative, "I hadn't heard that she's a woman," has all sorts of potentially hostile messages in it, including indignation because he was not informed earlier and surprise that anyone would hire a woman for a managerial position. Also, because the first word of the alternative is *I*, Fred's message might be that Larry could be in error, since Fred hadn't heard of it (Goody, 1978).

While the original utterance could be made hostile through voice inflection (emphasizing certain words), little or no hostility would be expressed if the utterance were said in a normal, polite tone of voice. Because the alternative is a statement rather than a question, it is potentially hostile on several fronts, even if it is said in a normal tone of voice. And it is the potential of hostility that a listener will sometimes respond to, thinking perhaps that the speaker is not very nice or is argumentative (Lyons, 1977; Elgin, 1980).

The question format has another advantage: It keeps the conversation going by offering the listener something to respond to. By using the question format, Fred is inviting Larry to respond. Larry can answer the question, supply further information, change the topic, or give a combination of responses. And as we see in utterance (4), Larry chooses to answer the question and supply more information.

Words and Structures Together

As communicators, we can say almost everything in a variety of ways. We can choose different words, and then put those words into different structures. By doing so, we communicate on at least two levels at once—an informational level and a social level. We know that some words are socially correct or polite, and some are not. Some structures are more polite or more threatening than others, giving the participants in a conversation a clue as to how each feels concerning what the other is saying and to what extent each wants the other to respond.

Putting these two aspects of language (the words and the structure) together creates a powerful weapon. Take something simple like the word *no*. The speaker's intended meaning may be no, but that is not always the word the speaker chooses to get that meaning across; in addition, lots of structures are available in which to place all those possible words. For example, a mother trying to keep the peace may say no to a toddler with the words *We'll see;* a father can say no to his sixteen-year-old son who wants to borrow the father's brand new Mercedes by saying, "Are you joking?" A worker may say no on the merits of a proposal suggested by his boss with "I'm not altogether sure about that," or "I may need more information before I could come to a conclusion"; and there is that emphatic expression, *no way!*

There are probably as many ways to say no as there are people. I have no doubt that new ways are being invented at this very moment. Just as we choose the words we want to say, we also create the structures in which to present them. And just as the words carry meaning, so do the structures in which we choose to place those words.

Level Two: The Way We Say Utterances

Once we have chosen the words and the structure to put them in, we must choose the way we want to say a sentence. And we have a lot of choices here, too.

I have divided level two into two categories, each representing a different way we can articulate a given sentence. The features of one category can work in conjunction with features from the other, but I will present them one at a time.

Voice Qualities

We use voice qualities to say a whole sentence or utterance in a certain way, and the different qualities we use can add meaning to the utterance. According to David Crystal and Randolph Quirk, the voice qualities are normal, whisper, breathiness, huskiness, creak, falsetto, and resonance (1964, pp. 37–41). A whisper often means that the utterance is a confidence, a secret not to be shared with those around the speaker and listener. A man might use falsetto to imitate a woman he is talking about, thereby showing the listener that it was the woman who said the words, and the man is simply repeating them. Resonance, or a deep, full, or rounded voice, could be used to make a show of importance.

These are just a few examples of the many ways we use voice qualities in face-to-face vocal communication. Voice qualities may not convey meaning in the way we are used to thinking of meaning, but they convey various types and levels of information to the listener. By doing so, they are very important to the overall understanding of an utterance (Crystal, 1982).

Prosodic Features

Prosodic features are the different ways we say a word or words within an utterance. For instance, we can emphasize a word and thereby make it stand out, or bring the pitch of our voice up at the end of the last word of an utterance to create a question. We can slip in pauses or pronounce one word precisely and exactly.

The basic prosodic features of our language are tone (fall to rise, rise to fall from word to word), tempo (how quickly or slowly we say a word), prominence (with how much gusto we say a word), pitch range (whether a word is said in a monotone or with exaggerated ups and downs), rhythmicality (whether a word flows naturally or is quick and spiky or staccato), and tension (whether the word is slurred or tense) (Crystal and Quirk, 1964).

More than one word in an utterance may be subject to a prosodic feature, and more than one prosodic feature may be used in any one utterance. For an example, let's look at the use of tone to create meaning. We will take one sentence and emphasize the tone of one word at a time. Since there are many aspects to tone, we will look at just one—tonic placement, or which word is emphasized in any given set of words.

John saw Mary in town. (Normal)
John saw Mary in *town*. (as opposed to somewhere else)
John saw *Mary* in town. (as opposed to someone else)

John saw Mary in town. (as opposed to someone else)
John *saw* Mary in town. (but didn't talk to her)

(Crystal, 1982; p. 116)

Each of the utterances contains the same words in the same order, yet the information they convey is not the same. The facts of the statement come from the arrangement of the words as well as the words chosen—John saw Mary in town. But very important (in some cases, equally important) information is conveyed through the selected use of tone.

Tone is only one of the prosodic features that contributes to meaning. Each feature makes a unique contribution to meaning depending on who uses the feature, how the feature is used, and in what situation the feature is used. All this information comes at us every time we listen to someone talk. We use these features in return, adding richness and depth to our communication.

Different uses of prosodic features and voice qualities can relay a lot of information to the listener and can help the listener understand how the speaker feels about the facts (bored or excited, impressed or doubtful). These features also can create sarcasm (by slurring the words while whispering) or any other tones of voice. They show the attitude of the speaker toward the information given in the words and structures, adding a whole new layer of meaning to the utterance.

They can also shift meanings within sentences by emphasizing certain aspects of the utterance and thereby adding to or emphasizing the meaning of a sentence. Compare the difference between *She* will have coffee and She will have *coffee*. In the first utterance, the person who is being referred to is being clarified, and in the second, the beverage in question is being clarified.

Level Three: The Way We Present Communication

The third level of spoken communication is nonverbal. When we speak, we gesture with our hands, our eyes and mouths, and our heads and shoulders, even the whole body. These gestures, when combined with what we say and how we say it, add a whole new dimension to the meaning of our utterances.

For example, how does a mother know if her small son is fibbing when she does not know for sure what the facts in the case are? She probably looks for the same telltale signs that my mom always looked for. First, is the child trying to hide his face? If he is, something is probably wrong. Second, how open are his eyelids? If the eyelids are half covering the eyes, there is something fishy. If the eyelids are high, the eyes are open, and he can look her full in the face, as if in surprise, then he is probably innocent.

The funny part about noticing a child's eyelid and head placement to determine whether or not the child is fibbing, is that it only works for a little while. Children soon learn how to get away with fibbing; they are able to flash those big, wide, innocent eyes right in your face and fib anyway.

You see, when we learn language as children, we learn all the parts of language. We learn not only what to say and how to say it, but how to present it in order to give the message we want. A raised eyebrow, a wrinkling of the nose, a lopsided grin are all a part of our language and our culture (Britton, 1970).

How often have we heard the term *shifty eyes*? The image that usually goes along with that term is of a disreputable man with a hat pulled low over his brow, his eyelids low, his eyes moving from side to side. He often has hunched shoulders, as if there is something secretive or furtive about his movements. And he has very little skin showing. His hands are gloved or in his pockets, the collar on his coat is turned up. He is hiding something! He is hiding information about himself by hiding the gestures that would give us clues as to how he feels about what he is saying.

We all use body movement in conversation to a greater or lesser extent. There is an old saying, "If you tied her hands together, she couldn't talk!" that describes someone who uses so many gestures they are intrinsic to her ability to communicate. On the other hand, there are those who use very few gestures indeed. Henry Kissinger, for example, can tell the funniest joke or describe whole scenes full of action and hardly move a muscle. My personal favorite is when a person raises one, just one, eyebrow. My sister can do that and I cannot, and it makes me jealous. When she does it, it is as if she is saying in the snootiest voice imaginable, "You don't say." It is so impolite, it is funny. I just love it.

These movements are all around us, giving us more information about the words spoken to us and the attitudes of the speaker. It would be to our advantage to pay more attention to them, to learn to listen not only with our ears, but, as much as we are able, with our eyes.

We could begin by becoming more aware of a person's body movements. Notice whether the speaker is relaxed and smiling or tense and hostile; whether he has a frown on his face and his eyes are beginning to squint. Is the speaker fiddling with a pencil as if he were ill at ease? Is he leaning forward, eyes alert on you, with a smile on his face? Knowing a person's attitude before you converse with him, or watching for changes while you are conversing, can be an added source of information concerning the speaker and what he is saying.

How Communication Changes for the Hearing-Impaired Person

So far, we have learned that language operates on three levels simultaneously. On two levels the signals are picked up by the ear, and on the third, by the eyes. All three levels are important for interpreting a message, which is everything one person tries to communicate to another.

We have already discussed how a hearing loss affects a person's ability to interpret speech. Now we are going to look at the ways hearing-impaired people can partially compensate for the loss of information conveyed by the three levels of language.

Missing Words

Word choice (the word or words a speaker chooses to use in a particular situation) is governed by a number of factors, including emotional stance. So when hearing-impaired people miss a word, when they do not hear it, they are in danger of losing not only the meaning behind the word, but the emotional content of the word. They do not just miss a word, but a complex interrelationship of meaning and thought; in other words, how the speaker thinks and feels about the subject.

Remember, we are dealing with spoken (rather than written) communication. We cannot pause, go back a couple of sentences, and figure it out. We have no time. We either understand or do not understand in seconds. There are few second chances.

Missing Structures

Do you remember how some structures are more polite than others? A big problem that a hard of hearing person might encounter is that, because she is missing some of the words, she may not be sure if someone has used a structure that is more aggressive or hostile than she believes the situation warrants.

Here is one scenario: You and a colleague are rushing to get a project done. You have finished your part of the project, but your colleague is bustling to finish his part. You notice that there is something you could do to help the colleague finish, but you are a little hesitant because you do not want to offend your colleague. So you say something such as, "Gee, I could do such and such for you, if you wouldn't mind?" The colleague, head down, looking at all the papers on his desk, could say, with a big sigh of relief, "If you *would . . .?*"

Now, the colleague meant to be polite back to you, and what the colleague actually said was polite, not only structurally (starting with *if* and creating a question), but in the way the utterance was said (with a sigh, indicating not just acceptance of your offer, but relief). Further, the fact that he was looking at all those papers could be interpreted as wonder that you would be willing to help him out of this mess, or even as shyness in accepting your help (Brown and Levinson, 1978).

But what if you heard, ". . . You would," which is not very polite, then the sigh might be interpreted as breathy mumbling, and the bowed head interpreted as concealment, to match what you thought you heard. Remember that our minds try to make meaning and make sense, make all the parts fit into a single message. All of a sudden, the whole situation has changed. The *if,* which softened and qualified the utterance, is missing and boom, you have a statement that is potentially nasty—"*You would* try and take over," "*You would* try and make me look bad." Then what do you do?

When in doubt, don't guess. Try, as best you can, to calm yourself. Say, very politely, "I didn't see your face, so I didn't understand what you just said. Could you please repeat it?" This is longer and more involved than a quick Excuse me?, or What?, or even Eve's Repeat, please?, but the reason you take time is because you want to be as polite as you can so your colleague can feel comfortable replying. After all, he might just have paid you a pretty big compliment. If you are brusque, abrupt, or accusatory, what is he going to think of you?

If you do not guess at meaning, if you slow down and try to make sure, you will always be the winner. Regardless of whether he was angry, as you thought he was, or polite, as he really was, your best bet is to be extra polite and find out for sure (Goody, 1978).

While misunderstanding can be distressing in any atmosphere, in the workplace where there is constant jockeying for position (status, respect, and recognition) between co-workers and members of a business community, the problem could have serious implications for hearing-impaired people. Their inability to interpret the politeness (or lack of) of an utterance could cause them to become insecure and/or victims of stress in an effort to hear every word and thereby circumvent the problem.

Either insecurity or stress by itself could greatly affect job performance. It can become a vicious circle. When the hearing-impaired person is comfortable with explaining what might have been missed or misinterpreted, and pleasantly asks for repetition or clarification, that vicious circle often can be broken. Such tactics can even enhance self-respect and, in turn, garner the respect of others.

As we found out earlier, the way we say words can give clues to both meaning and emotional content, but this may be even harder for hearing-impaired people to hear than the words themselves. The use of different voice qualities and prosodic features is often very small or subtle. Since hearing-impaired people usually focus their attention on just the words, they are more likely to miss the special way a speaker emphasizes a word or sentence.

As a result, hearing-impaired people miss the feelings or attitudes the speaker has toward the topic of conversation. Those feelings and attitudes reveal information both about the topic and the speaker. When that information is missed, it can be difficult (or impossible) to tell if the speaker was being polite, snide, encouraging, sarcastic, happy, or downright hostile. Can you imagine trying to move up the corporate ladder without being able to interpret a speaker's attitudes and feelings? If you have been there, you know how tough it is. And if you have not been there, count yourself very fortunate.

You may be wondering if anything can be done about this problem. The answer is yes. The solutions are not substitutes for what is missing, but they will at least give you a fighting chance.

Finding Solutions

The first thing you can do is to pay more attention to the way a person says something. As some people lose their hearing, they tend to focus more and more attention on catching all the words. This means they will focus their eyes harder and harder on just the mouth and focus their attention harder and harder on interpreting just the words. As you have seen, while the words are certainly important to meaning, they contain within them only one part of the potential meaning of any particular utterance. By ignoring all the other available signals and concentrating on the words alone, hearing-impaired people actually may be reducing their chances of correctly interpreting the message rather than increasing them.

So what do they do? Stop concentrating on the words? No, of course not. But there is a difference between focusing one's whole attention on the words and being more aware of them. By using prediction (see chapter 7), hearing-impaired listeners will be able to anticipate better what the next words will be, and thereby relieve some of the pressure of focusing only on the words in order to catch them all. This leaves some room to direct attention to the features of conversation that cannot be predicted; in other words, voice qualities, prosodic features, gesture, and movement.

By giving some attention to the way people say words and how they present them, hearing-impaired listeners will be able to pick up many of the emotional and informational aspects of the conversation that they may have been missing. Often (although not always) the second and third levels of language (voice quality and body motion) echo each other, so if listeners miss one, they can sometimes pick it up from the other. And both levels two and three are echoed in level one, through the speaker's choice of words and structures (Birdwhistell, 1970).

Let's examine this closer. Suppose you are talking with your friend Linda. She knows you normally do not like to go shopping, but she needs to purchase a new pair of running shoes. She asks, "Would you like to go with me?" She does not know that you need a new sweat suit and that you would much prefer going shopping with her to going alone.

You answer, "Yes, I'd like that very much," with so much enthusiasm that Linda, who is expecting a negative reply, is startled. Her head jerks as she quickly looks you full in the face, her eyes widen, her eyebrows go up, and then she smiles. Her surprise and delight will show in her voice. It will probably be a little louder and a little higher pitched than usual because of her excitement. And her reply is "*Really?* That's *great!*"

The repetitiveness of language is a very important concept. Shannon's communication theory (see chapter 7) included the idea that a message that is repeated will be more likely to be understood than a message that is not repeated. Well, that is certainly logical. We usually think of repetition as saying the message again, but there is another aspect of repetition, and it is contained in the three levels of spoken language.

Remember that short-term memory and the mind have only seconds to interpret a spoken message, and that we seldom, if ever, get a second chance? Then how is it possible for us to understand something as complex and as fleeting as spoken language? Part of the answer is that the meaning (both factual and emotional) of the spoken message is given in at least three ways: by the words and structures we choose, by the way we choose to say an utterance, and by the way we present the utterance. In other words, the message is repeated, but it is repeated on each level simultaneously (Crystal and Quirk, 1964).

We learn how to interpret the second and third levels of spoken communication by paying attention to them. "Ah," you say, "It can't be that easy!" Well, you are right. Learning to predict so you can pay more attention to the other aspects of language is not all that easy. You need to practice. And learning to watch and listen for the second- and third-level aspects of language is not easy, either. That takes practice, too. But you've had a lot of practice in your life interpreting what voice qualities and gesture mean. Really!

You see, interpreting spoken communication on all its levels is a part of our culture. We do not need to read a book to know that a shrug combined with raised eyebrows means "I don't know." We know what that gesture means just as surely as we know what the word *cat* means. It is already a part of our vocabulary. We know how to talk politely, use polite structures and words and gestures. And we know what is not polite (Brown and Levinson, 1978).

When David Crystal (1982) talked about linguistic disabilities, he pointed out that we learn the prosodic aspects of speech at a very early age indeed. In fact, he said, "Certainly by 12 months [of age], in most children, [some] tone units . . . are well established as a means of organizing speech—whether the speech be 'one word sentences' or an unintelligible 'jargon' " (p. 117). In other words, a one-year-old uses second-level communication skills even though she does not even know the words to attach to those features.

If you are a parent, you've probably seen this. Your youngster may have had a vocabulary of only twenty words or so, but he or she had many ways to say each of those words. Each different way he or she said the word meant something different. For example, two of the most versatile words are *no* and *Mommy*. *No* can mean any of the following: "I didn't do that, really truly," "I won't do that, no matter what," "I really don't think so," "I'd rather not," or "This is not at all what I intended." *Mommy* runs the gamut from "Help!" "How could you?" "Why won't you?" "Where are you?" "Why can't I?" to "I love you." Ah, communication, it's great!

All of us have the capability to understand when a structure or a word or a voice quality or prosodic feature or gesture is polite or hostile, creates a question or a statement, or conveys a hundred other meanings. The goal is to become more aware of the features and to use them to your advantage.

Becoming more aware of the levels and features of spoken American English will greatly assist hearing-impaired people in understanding conversation. Still, there will be times when they are just not sure what was said or what the tenor or emotional thrust of an utterance was. This is true for people with normal hearing, as well, but it is a more frequent problem for those who are hearing impaired. The solution to this problem is the same for people with a hearing loss as for people who have normal hearing, and that is socially correct, old-fashioned courtesy in its most formal usage.

For the first (and next-to-the-last) time, my mother and I would like to strongly recommend the book *Miss Manners' Guide to Excruciatingly Correct Behavior* by Judith Martin (1982). That's right, Miss Manners. We would also recommend you begin reading her syndicated column in your local newspaper. Why? The answer is simple—if you are not sure you understood someone correctly (on all levels) and you feel that this person's utterance was potentially unpleasant or hostile, you have three courses of action.

1. Get angry. Whip around to face the speaker and say in a loud, threatening manner, "What did you say?" While this can, under certain circumstances, be effective, most of the time it is not.

   What if you completely misunderstood the speaker? Then you may have given yourself the reputation of being, at best, short-tempered and, at worst, a mean old grouch! What if your suspicions were correct? The speaker will probably evade the whole issue by saying, "I wasn't talking to/about you," or "Nothing, nothing at all."

The point is to give the speaker a lesson in politeness while at the same time making clear that, hearing loss notwithstanding, you are not to be trifled with. And you cannot do that unless you are sure of what was said.

2. Ignore the whole thing and do not respond at all. Again, while there are situations that should be ignored, when the most polite thing you can do is pretend something was never done or said, this usually is not one of them. By ignoring the utterance, you have put yourself at a linguistic disadvantage. You are admitting that the speaker has control of the language, and therefore, the situation.

   The world contains many unkind people who understand this basic fact and who are more than ready to trade on the power they gain through abusive language or innuendo, in the hopes that their victim will do just what solution two indicates—nothing.

3. Stop dead in your tracks, slowly turn to face the speaker, put on a partially serious, partially inquiring expression and say, "Excuse me, but I didn't quite catch that. Would you mind repeating it for me?" Then just look at the person. Try not to have a hostile expression on your face, for that would defeat your purpose. Open and innocent and interested, if you can manage it, serves very well. I think of it as a cross between a ten-year-old boy asking for a piece of candy and an eager college student waiting for words of wisdom from her favorite professor.

   What can the speaker do? If the utterance really was innocent, he will probably tell you what he said. When this happens, you will want to listen to the speaker until he finishes and then show an interest in what he repeated to you by commenting on it or by taking the time to join in conversation for a moment or two. If the utterance was as nasty as you thought it was, then the speaker will probably not dare repeat it. Any other person who happened to hear the utterance will be watching, knowing the speaker has put himself in a heck of a jam, and since you have demonstrated your skill in dealing with this nasty-minded speaker, the other listener will not want any part of it.

The worst case scenario is that the speaker did say something nasty and repeats it again at your request. At this point you are no better or worse off than if you had heard the comment in the first place, and since you now know, without a doubt, what was said, you can act accordingly.

You have taken control of the situation. You have shown yourself to be reasonable, which, in the case of the innocent speaker, will allow you to make the point that you are interested in what he has to say. It also allows you to show that you are a courteous person who is easy to talk to. In the case of the nasty speaker, you have shown yourself to be a formidable speaker yourself, someone who is courteous but firm and well aware of the social niceties of language and the social standards of the community. It puts you in control, so much so, that if the nasty speaker does not or cannot say anything, you can let him off the hook with something like, "Well, I guess it's time we get back to work, don't you think?" If he still cannot respond, you can look him in the eye one more time (and if you can do it, raise one eyebrow), and say, "Just so." Then turn and go back to whatever it was you were doing.

Being polite, knowing that you are socially correct, goes beyond maintaining the upper hand in nasty situations. These social skills can give you confidence in all facets of your life and help you feel more comfortable communicating with a variety of people. The more comfortable and relaxed you are, the better you will understand what is being said. We recommend *Miss Manners*, Judith Martin, for help in learning these politeness strategies.

Linguistic nastiness comes in many forms and is used by many different types of people for many different reasons. All-out attacks, however, come in recognizable patterns and you can learn not only to recognize these attacks but how to gracefully and appropriately defend yourself. For just how to do this, I recommend Suzette Haden Elgin's book *The Gentle Art of Verbal Self-Defense* (1980). Elgin is an applied psycholinguist and an associate professor of linguistics at San Diego State University. In this excellent book she has created a course for recognizing verbal attacks and replying to them. I found this easy-to-read, step-by-step book to be a real eye-opener and almost immediately useful. If you feel you are losing control in conversations with certain people, if talking with this or that person always makes you feel inadequate or stupid or down-right puzzled, then give this book a try.

I have often wondered why (along with Elgin), if linguistic nastiness is so prevalent, we do not have mandatory classes in grade school, high school, and college to teach people how to deal with it. The good news is that politeness has not disappeared altogether. By better understanding the nature of spoken communication, as well as learning how to frame polite questions and, when necessary, how to respond to linguistic nastiness, we can more effectively take control and defuse potentially explosive, emotionally costly situations.

Part Three
Communication

Eleven

The Basics of Communicating with a Hard of Hearing Person

Trying to communicate with a person who is hard of hearing can be frustrating, puzzling, or just downright difficult. Solid, loving relationships are built on good communication (sharing experiences, information, and feelings), and when someone loses the ability to communicate, to any degree, a strain is put on the relationship.

We have looked at the problems people who suffer a hearing loss experience and how this loss can affect their lives, but this is really only half the story. It takes two to communicate effectively; both parties must work hard at saying what they mean to say in such a way that the other can understand it. In addition, they both must work hard at listening, trying to understand correctly and fully the content of the message. If both speakers are not participating in the communication process effectively, the results can strain the relationship, change dynamics of the relationship, and potentially destroy the relationship.

The purpose of this chapter is to give hearing readers some insights into what they can do to foster good communication with a hard of hearing person. We will also talk about the things we have learned in our family in the hopes that they will help others find ways of communicating more effectively.

We are conscious of the fact that what works for us may not work for others; we also know that not all people are going to have the same problems. So, when reading this section, please try to keep in mind that our solutions may have to be modified to fit individual situations. We do not have all the answers; human relationships defy almost any single definition or black and white analysis.

The particular problems you and your hearing-impaired family member(s), friends, or clients are having will depend greatly on the extent of their hearing loss, the type of hearing loss they have suffered, and the kinds of hearing aids and assistive devices they are using.

Physical Surroundings

In chapter 3 Eve explained some of the ways hearing-impaired people can arrange their surroundings to their advantage. An assertive hard of hearing person will direct a hearing person to a room or a special chair to take advantage of the available lighting and to minimize background noise. Hearing people also should be aware of the importance of the surroundings to make communication easier for everyone. Let's look at some of the ways to improve the communication setting.

Line of Sight

It took me years to understand the importance of a clear line of sight, but once I did, oh, what a difference it made! When Eve's hearing loss was mild I could shout for her or call her name behind her back and she would respond just like always. As her hearing dropped, sometimes she would reply, and sometimes she wouldn't. Since the technique still worked some of the time, I continued talking to her behind her back and expecting her to understand me. Big mistake.

The result was I became confused because sometimes she responded and sometimes she didn't. I even got angry when I thought (completely incorrectly) that she was ignoring me. When my mom didn't seem to get what I said, I would get upset that she hadn't understood me. It would have been so much better for both of us had I learned and used this very simple rule: If she can't see me, she can't hear me.

The best thing you can do for your hearing-impaired friend or family member is to remember this rule. Everything else— lighting, pronunciation, and topic selection—depends on this one simple rule. In order to make it work, this rule has to be followed all of the time. If you want to talk to your father, who is hearing-impaired, then go find him, don't shout from room to room.

However, this advice to go find the person must be tempered with some common sense. One thing you will want to remember is to never walk up behind a hearing-impaired person who is engrossed in a task. We hearing people need to understand that, in many cases, hearing-impaired people cannot (1) hear that we have moved from our last position, (2) hear that we have walked toward their position, or (3) hear that we have walked up behind them.

Our mind takes care of all these little details for us, even while we are busy. It keeps tabs on our surroundings for us and allows us to concentrate on tasks at hand, secure in the knowledge that we will be warned when we are about to be interrupted. But many hard of hearing people have lost the ability to keep track of those movements, and severely hard of hearing people cannot hear footsteps at all. You can give someone quite a bad scare by sneaking up on them. (I know, from your perspective you weren't sneaking, but from their point of view, that may be exactly what you did.)

My mom is pretty resourceful and she has some creative ways of getting around not being able to hear footsteps. I can remember a particularly bright, warm spring morning when Mom and I sat talking over a second cup of coffee. At that time she could still hear face-to-face communication fairly well with the help of two hearing aids.

"Oh," she said, breaking into the conversation. "I've got to get Bill's breakfast finished. He's just about to come downstairs."

I stared at her, wondering if she had perfected mindreading. I knew that he was up and about because I could hear him moving around upstairs, but how on earth did she know?

"Did you *hear* him?" I asked her, wondering what was going on.

She laughed. "No, of course not. I can smell his after-shave."

By golly, she was right. I sniffed, and sure enough, the smell of the after-shave he has used all his adult life was there, very faint.

"The fan system on the furnace circulates the air," Mom explained. "So the smell comes right through the air ducts." She is one smart cookie, my mom.

Unfortunately, we normally have to rely on our hearing to tell us if someone we cannot see is coming our way. So how do we approach hard of hearing people when they cannot see us? My solution is to wait in doorways. After I first enter the house, if Mom is not aware I am there and not expecting me, I look around to find her. Then I wait in the doorway or hall or on the basement stairs for her to notice me. The trick is to wait as far away as I can and still be in her line of sight. I must say, there are times when I feel like bringing a book along to enliven the wait, but for the most part, she turns and sees me in a minute or so. Another solution is to flash the lights on and off when you walk into a room. This will be sure to alert the hearing-impaired person to your presence.

In any event, it is no use bemoaning the fact that a hearing-impaired person can no longer hear your step or understand you when you call. Just remember the rule: If a person with a hearing loss cannot see you, he or she cannot hear you.

Lighting

Try never to put your back to the available light source. By back-lighting your body, you make it very difficult for hearing-impaired people to pick up visual cues from your face. The better they can see you, the better they will be able to hear you.

Background Noise

Background noise is very detrimental to hard of hearing people. Consider that, under ideal conditions, they retain only a percentage of their ability to hear and their hearing aids amplify most sounds unselectively, particularly mechanical sounds. To hearing people, the sound of a fan or a truck going by is an annoyance. But to hard of hearing people, it can be a disaster. What slender hold they had on a conversation can be completely wiped out, especially if they are wearing hearing aids. Everyday sounds can potentially overwhelm them and make it utterly impossible for them to maintain the conversation.

Never try to hold a prolonged or important conversation with a hearing-impaired person when you are around equipment or machine noises. Taboo places include kitchens, basements, stores, automobiles, many office and factory areas, or any place where there are poor acoustics and/or background noises. Listen a moment and you can determine the level of background noise—Can you hear cars going by? Is there canned music playing in the background? Are others talking near you, as in a restaurant situation?

The rule of thumb I use is this: If I can easily identify the sounds, then they are potentially loud enough to interfere with my mother's hearing aid and implant processor and make it difficult for her to hear. So that is not the time or place to hold an in-depth conversation.

If you need to have an important or long conversation with a hard of hearing person, then get to a controlled or controllable environment, such as a house, apartment, or conference room. Sometimes it is as simple as moving away from a group of people or stepping out on a quiet terrace, but many times it takes much thought and planning.

Even if you are in a perfectly controlled environment, momentary noises can cause the hearing-impaired person to be swamped with electronic garbage. A heavy truck may go by, an airplane may fly overhead; all sorts of noises intrude on us daily. If this happens when I am talking, I have learned to stop and wait for the noise to go away. I find this very hard to do because I want to continue with what I am saying, but I have learned the hard way that continuing is pointless. I will just have to repeat it all over again when the noise is gone, and it frustrates my mom when she tries to hear through these noises, so no one gets anywhere. Once you get used to it, the wait is not really so bad. I spend the time getting my thoughts in order or just looking about.

You do not need to be as careful with casual conversations, but you should still be aware that environmental sounds can frustrate both you and the hearing-impaired person. So, try to be considerate of his or her needs. And of course, a smile, a wave, and a quick hello said directly at the hard of hearing person can be understood in the middle of a grand slam home run in Dodger stadium, so do not be afraid to let people know you notice them and wish them well. Communication can be simple, short, and sweet as well as lengthy and complicated, but it all counts. It is all important to each of us.

Acoustics

As with background sound, the acoustics of a room or building can potentially cause havoc for a hard of hearing person. A short list of the acoustically worst places includes all doctors' and dentists' examining and work rooms, large offices, kitchens, basements, factories, gyms, showers, bathrooms, and classrooms. The causes of bad acoustics are tile and/or concrete walls or floors; lack of carpeting, drapes, or stuffed or plush furnishings; and little or no acoustical ceiling tiles.

Quick conversations can be held in most places as long as you realize the necessity of speaking a bit more clearly to overcome the deficiencies in acoustics. However, if the conversation turns serious or if you know you will engage in a lengthy discussion, you might want to suggest moving to more comfortable surroundings, such as a plush office, boardroom, or a living room where the hard of hearing person will have less trouble following your speech.

Hearing Aids and Assistive Devices

It is the hearing impaired person's job to let you know if she is wearing a hearing aid or cochlear implant processor. She should also inform you of what voice qualities are comfortable for her. It is your job to listen carefully to what she says regarding her needs and to try, as much as possible, to meet them. You might even try a couple of test sentences to adjust the range of your voice to best interact with the hearing aids. After that it is simply a matter of remembering how loudly and how distinctly to talk to that particular person.

Noticing whether or not a person is wearing hearing aids is a shared responsibility. If the hearing-impaired person realizes you are trying to talk to her, but she is not wearing aids, she might say to you, "I'm sorry but I don't have my hearing aids in." She should then let you know when you can communicate. But many times the hard of hearing person will not even know you are trying to talk to her. For example, suppose you are getting dressed after a workout at your club. You turn to the hard of hearing person next to you and comment on the new equipment. Now, it is entirely possible that she will completely ignore you. Because of the electronic nature of hearing aids and processors, your friend probably will put them on after she is completely dressed and her hair is dry to make sure the aids do not come in contact with wet ears or damp hair. She also wants to avoid knocking the aids off inadvertently while putting on a t-shirt or sweater.

My mother never wears her cochlear implant processor while gardening because all of the bending down and mucking about in the bushes may dislodge it. I know of other people who take off their hearing aids every now and then at work to give their ears a rest. Some hearing aids fit very snugly inside the ears; some fit so snugly that they are airtight, so the insides of the ears become moist and clammy. Sometimes people just need a respite from the constant drone of noise. In fact, there are hundreds of reasons why a person might wish to take off her hearing aids. So if the hard of hearing person does not respond, look for the hearing aids. Then use your judgment concerning whether or not to wait for her to put them on voluntarily or to signal that you would like or need to talk to her.

Communication Techniques

Once you have the setting under control, you may need to make some changes in the way you speak. This will depend on the extent of the person's hearing loss and whether or not that person has any other problems that will affect the ability to understand on that particular day at that particular moment. But even if the hearing-impaired person is having no trouble hearing you under controlled conditions at this point in time, you might consider beginning to practice deliberate speech anyway. Unfortunately, many people who are hard of hearing lose more of their hearing as time goes on. If you start to change your speech habits now, then you have a much better chance of maintaining the quality of your conversations for a longer time.

Face Front

The easiest thing you can do is to face the listener directly, with the available light shining in your face. I know that is a bit uncomfortable when you are outside on a sunny day, but it is such an immense help to the hard of hearing person that her ability to understand what you are saying more than makes up for it.

At the same time, you must remember to *not* put your hand in front of your face or mouth while you talk. In addition, men who are not clean-shaven should remember to keep their moustaches and/or beards neatly trimmed so that their lips are clearly visible.

Speak Up and Slow Down

You may need to change the pace and loudness of your speech to make yourself more easily understood. More is involved here than just talking loudly, so let's go through it one step at a time.

Loudness

In a way loudness is the easiest variable to change, but it has the potential of getting you into trouble, too. First of all, the hearing-impaired person may not need you to speak louder at all. His hearing aids may already be giving him enough volume. If you are in doubt, ask, "Do you need me to speak more loudly?" If he replies yes, then you may encounter a second problem. When many people speak more loudly, they raise the pitch of their voices. In some cases, this may be good for the listener, but it is almost always bad for the speaker. You see, raising the pitch of your voice, especially for a long period of time, can make your throat very sore.

What you want to try to do is speak at the same pitch, just more loudly. You do this by relaxing your throat and putting more air through it, giving your voice more force without changing pitch. People who lecture have learned to do this, and it may help you to pretend you are talking to a small group of people until you get the hang of it. It just takes a little practice.

Length

Sometimes hearing people have a tendency to abbreviate their conversation when talking with hard of hearing people. Instead of talking in sentences, as they would for people without hearing problems, they will talk in a sort of shorthand of words and phrases. They do this with the mistaken thought that the fewer words hard of hearing people have to listen for, the more words they are likely to get. But this is not normally the case.

Meaning in language does not just come from the words we speak, but from the structures into which we put those words. Just think of all the different ways there are to say no, depending on the situation we happen to be in—"No, you can't." "That's not a good idea." "We'll see." "I wouldn't do that if I were you." "I'm not sure I agree." Each of these no's means something a little different, and by shorthanding all of them to no, the differences in structure and meaning would be lost.

Another problem with shorthanding is that hearing-impaired people need every little bit of information available within the language to have a chance of getting meaning. They know the structures of their language; they have been using them properly for years. They are expecting to get those structures back, actively listening for them and for the clues to meaning that they hold.

Speed

As you can see, the structure is very important. It lends a cadence to speech. If you slow down your speech to accommodate a hard of hearing person, then you must do so in such a way that those cadences or rhythms remain intact. This is not as hard as it sounds. What you are trying to do is slow down but still have the speech sound natural. Let's take this sentence for example:

Waking up is impossible without a cup of coffee.

Now that you have read it, try saying it out loud, as you would in a normal conversation. Go ahead, do it. Good. Now do it again, but listen to how you put the words together, where you run one word into the next, and where you pause. You may have to say it a couple of times to hear everything that's going on. When I say it out loud, it comes out something like this:

Wakingup-s im poss-able wi-thout-a cu-pa coffee.

As you can see, when something is written we have lots of breaks, but when it is spoken we tend to run sounds together. All you need to do is be a little more aware of how you naturally talk and then make all the breaks between words and phrases a little clearer. For example, when talking with my mother I might say the sentence like this:

Waking up-s im-poss-able without a-cup of-coffee.

There is really not a lot of difference between the two spoken sentences. I just cleaned up my pronunciation and slowed down a bit. In the places where there was a little pause, I put a bigger pause. And where there was a big pause, I put a bigger pause. But the rhythm, the cadence of the sentence, is essentially the same.

Pronunciation

Pronunciation is the big problem. Except for professional stage actors, most of us talk as though we have a mouthful of mush. If you live with a person who has any kind of a hearing problem, then now is the time to start cleaning up your speech. And if you cannot do it alone, join a local theater group and take acting lessons. I am not kidding. You will learn to enunciate, vocalize, project, and control pitch, all the things you may have to learn to keep the lines of communication open between you and a person who is losing her hearing.

With pronunciation, you are not trying to change everything about the way you talk, you are just trying to be more careful. Pronounce words as if you are reading them, which means being especially careful to try and finish words off, such as saying the *r* in *other* and the *th* in *both*. The goal is to give the hearing-impaired person all the information you possibly can by deliberately shaping your words. The more information the person has to work with, the more likely it is he or she will understand what you are saying.

When you talk with people who are hard of hearing, you need to help them get all they can from the words (by pronouncing them clearly) and the structures (by keeping the rhythms of speech intact) while you adjust the speed and loudness of your speech. It is a little like patting your head and rubbing your stomach at the same time, but you can learn how to do it. And what a difference it makes.

Gestures

With a little bit of practice, you can augment your speech with common, everyday movements that will significantly help the hard of hearing person understand what you are saying. I am talking about very simple gestures that will assist the hard of hearing person. Although American Sign Language (ASL) is a truly wonderful language that has made communication accessible to many deaf people, for most older hearing-impaired people it is not the answer.

First of all, ASL is a language in and of itself; it is not just signed speech. ASL has its own grammar and syntax. Learning ASL is like learning a foreign language, which is difficult for many of us. But the biggest problem for most people is that none of their friends or family know how to sign. Neither do their doctors or lawyers or the bank tellers or grocery clerks. So, while ASL is a logical, viable alternative for some people, for many it is not.

Gestures, however, are native to all of us. Each language has a set of gestures that go along with it, and we all know the meaning of most of them. Point at your temple and move your finger in a circle, and most any American-born person will interpret the message as "crazy person." Thumbs up means "Yes!" or "Well done!"

These signals can reinforce the meanings of your words, giving the hard of hearing person extra, sometimes vital, information. For example, if you are talking about the price of a car that you wish to buy, and the car costs twelve thousand dollars, when you say, "twelve thousand dollars" you might also signal with your fingers a one, then a two. If your response to a question is "I don't know," you could also lift your hands and shrug your shoulders. We can combine many body and facial movements a hundred different ways that will help show the listener what we are saying, giving vital clues to words or to the meaning of entire sentences.

Try to use your body more expressively, to exaggerate the tilt of your head, the widening of your eyes. You might want to pretend you are playing a mild game of charades. The information you communicate with your body could well make the difference between a hard of hearing person understanding you or becoming completely lost.

A word or two of warning—gestures are as individual and cultural as slang. An innocent and acceptable gesture in American English might be an obscene gesture in Australian English. When communicating with a non-American, it is sometimes safest to keep gestures to a minimum.

Keeping Track of the Topic

When a hard of hearing person is involved in a conversation, he often gets only little bits and pieces of the words and must construct meaning through a series of guesses. Obviously, there are going to be quite a few times when that person guesses incorrectly. The most likely place in a conversation for this to happen is at a change of topic. This is because the hearing-impaired person has no way of guessing what the new topic might be, so is often conversationally left in the dust.

In a two-way conversation, you need to remember to warn the listener when you change the topic. Depending on the severity of his or her hearing impairment, this warning can be handled much the way it is with a hearing person, by saying something such as, "By the way, did you know that . . ." or "And speaking of movies, did you happen to see. . . ." We do this often when we change the subject in conversations with people who have normal hearing. We just need to try to remember to do it all the time with those who are hard of hearing.

For those people with more severe hearing problems, you might just come right out and say, "This is a change of topic," or "I'm changing the topic now." Subtlety in this situation will not win awards or get results. Just jump right up there and tell them what is happening, and you will find they will track right along with you.

When a person is severely hearing impaired, or less impaired but involved in a group conversation (a total of three or more people talking together), then you might want to work out a hand signal for the person to use when he or she has lost the topic. As Eve said in chapter 4, when she loses track of the topic, she makes a *T* with her hands, just like a football player does when asking for time out.

This is how it works for us: Eve will look toward one of the people who is not talking, put a questioning look on her face (raised eyebrows) and signal *T* with her hands. This means, "I've lost the topic. What is it?" The person will give her a brief answer, perhaps the subject of the conversation or the name of the person being talked about along with a key phrase, something to clue her in to the topic. Then she usually smiles and nods her head, and she is back into the flow.

This technique is very unobtrusive, and it allows the hard of hearing person to control the assistance he or she gets, which is very important. After all, how would you like it if someone distracted you from a conversation every five minutes and said, "Now, are you getting all this, dear?" You see, we cannot always know when hard of hearing people are not "getting it," so we have to let them tell us. It may be that they are tired and they are not listening for a couple of minutes on purpose, just to get a rest. So try to relax, let the conversation go where it will, and keep an eye out for signals from the hearing-impaired person.

The trick is to have some sort of system that works for you and is understood between you and the hard of hearing person, and then let him or her cue you. That way you will all get the most enjoyment possible out of the conversation.

Conversation Flow and Interrupting

Another problem hard of hearing people have with conversations involving more than two people is that they have trouble telling when a person has finished speaking.

Conversations are, in a way, lessons in politeness; each person in a conversational group waits his turn before speaking. The clues that tell us the difference between the speaker pausing for a second or two and the speaker relinquishing control to another speaker are very subtle. They involve pitch, eye contact, and body movement, as well as meaning (or word) clues. Even among those with perfect hearing, you will notice that people will often pause a moment before becoming the next speaker, just to make sure that the first speaker has finished. That is because the vocal and nonvocal signals are not often absolutely clear and direct (Bennett, 1976; Goody, 1978).

Hearing-impaired people have trouble because in addition to not getting any subtle verbal cues, they probably are missing the nonverbal cues as well. They expend so much, if not all, of their awareness on making basic meaning, on watching and listening for all of the spoken meaning cues, that they cannot do this and spare any attention for the more subtle shifts of language. As a result, the cues for conversation breaks tend to go right by them. When this happens, hearing-impaired people are left with one of two choices—say nothing or interrupt.

If a hearing-impaired person is unsure when it is or is not polite to take her turn speaking, she will sometimes just not try at all. Perhaps she has been criticized too often or harshly for interrupting, or perhaps she is afraid of appearing rude or stupid. Whatever the case, she is afraid of causing any further damage to the relationships built and sustained by conversation. Why *further* damage? Because it is the hearing impairment that made communication difficult in the first place.

I am not saying that this perception is fair, or even true. Certainly, no one is at fault. No one person ever is, when it comes to communication. It is no one's fault that someone loses hearing. But look at it from that person's perspective—in her view, everything is the same except her. No one else has changed, she has. And it is not just a broken leg that might be keeping the family from a camping trip. This is forever.

On the other hand, if the hard of hearing person constantly interrupts, then the hearing person may think that she is just a rude person and may cease to hold conversations with her. That is not a viable solution either, because you end up throwing away what could be a very rich, loving relationship.

Again, the key to solving the problem rests in recognizing that the problem exists, that it is a real, physical problem (not a character flaw). Then learn to work around that problem. Just as in the case of hand signals to cue a lost topic, some sort of signal arrangement can easily be worked out to cue the hearing-impaired person when there has been a conversation break to allow a shift from one speaker to another.

My mother has a tendency to raise her index finger, sort of an imitation of a person in a classroom holding up her hand for a turn to speak. While she is doing this, as in the change of topic cue, she will look at someone in the conversation group, either the immediate speaker or a listener, for an answer. What she is silently asking is, "Can I speak now?" All I have to do is nod yes or no, and she can take it from there.

"Repeat, Please"

When my mother misses a few words in a conversation, she says, "Repeat, please." Most of the time this works very well since she asks for the repeat as soon as she realizes she didn't understand what was said. However, sometimes just saying the words over again does not work. This can be frustrating (to say the least) for both of us. I keep saying the words, and she keeps misunderstanding the words. There is a reason for this. Let me explain.

Each of us carries in our heads our own world view. Each of us has had different life experiences—different childhoods, adolescences, adulthoods—and we are the sum total of all our unique thoughts and experiences. Language is our attempt to overcome our differences and create communication between all people who share a language, regardless of each individual's personal experiences or knowledge. Considering the vast differences that we are trying to overcome, language works pretty darn well. But it is not perfect.

A linguistic community (a group of people who share the same language) agrees upon basic structures for language and the basic meanings of the words used in that language. But because each of us is different, a great potential exists for one person to misunderstand what another person feels is perfectly clear. ("Well, I know what I meant.") An example of this occurs when one person in a conversation group works in a totally different field from the others.

For instance, one of the tenants at the apartment complex where I used to live had a party in the common courtyard. He invited a bunch of his co-workers over for a barbecue. My apartment was on the courtyard, so I listened to a bit of their conversation. They might as well have been speaking German, for all I understood them. You see, they were all doctors in residency at the local Veteran's Administration medical center. They knew the meanings to words I simply do not know. They were talking "doctor talk," a sublanguage of English that I never studied. There are hundreds of sublanguages—each profession has its own vocabulary (such as computerese). We can recognize the connecting words like *and* and *or*, and some of the words that the parent language and sublanguage have in common, but even the words that are common to both do not necessarily carry the same meaning. To a doctor working in a hospital, a *bed* is somewhere to put or find a patient. To me, a bed is something to sleep in.

Our personal world view creates in each of us a sort of sublanguage or personal code for words, codes not shared by the general community. For example, if someone said to you, "I have a dog," what would you think of? Well, you probably would not think of the dictionary definition. Like me, you probably think of one or several particular dogs that you have known.

Now the problem with communication is that everyone who hears the statement, "I have a dog," probably pictures a different dog, depending upon personal experience or world view. Every word we hear is made meaningful to us by our interpretation of that word through our personal world view. That is one way that two speakers talking the same dialect of the same sublanguage of the same language can completely misunderstand one another.

The person who said "I have a dog" may have meant toy poodle and the person who was listening might have seen in their mind English sheepdog.

When the mind gets hold of what it considers to be the meaning behind the word, it resists giving up that meaning. Unless we are told straight out "I meant a toy poodle," we will continue to think of "English sheepdog," even when it starts to get silly. For example, if our friend tells us about his new dog but does not tell us what kind of dog it is, and then relates a story of how this dog loves to sit in people's laps and sleep with him, our mental picture of a fully grown English sheepdog popping into a grandmother's lap or jumping into and busting a bed could start us chuckling. We might even realize at this point we do not really know what kind of dog our friend has because what he is telling us about the dog, coupled with our picture of what we believe the dog to be, is starting to get a little weird.

The mind is trying to make meaning. To do so, it takes what it thought it heard, translates that into its world view, and uses this to create meaning. When the mind feels it has been successful at all these mental gymnastics, it does not really want to worry about it any more. It has done its job and created meaning, so it prepares for the next bit of sound to transform that into meaning. In order to be prepared for the next piece of work it must do, the mind holds on to its first meaningful impression, regardless of whether or not it is right.

This is why, especially when talking to a hearing-impaired person, you need to learn to say things differently if you are not going to be misunderstood. Put another way, if you pronounced it as best you could two or three times and the hearing-impaired person still did not get it, then try saying the phrase differently.

New Words, New Chances

When you communicate with someone who is hard of hearing, you may need to get used to finding alternative ways of saying things. If I have twice asked my mom, "Are you going out on the boat today?" and her reply was at first a look of confusion and then something off the wall, such as, "Am I working on the books today?" then I know she has taken what she could understand of the words I said, plunked them into her world view, and ended up with something completely unlike anything I had intended to communicate. She has made meaning, perhaps not the meaning I wanted her to make, but it *is* meaning. If I repeat yet again, "No, I said, 'Are you going out on the boat today?'" then all she is probably going to hear are the bits and pieces that confirm she had the right meaning in the first place. Her mind is working along these lines: "Yes, yes. I heard that the first time. Now what's the next bit?" Do not blame the hearing-impaired person because this happens to all of us. And for heavens sake, do not get mad. It is nobody's fault. Her mind did its job (made meaning from what it thought it heard) and now confirms the meaning by hearing the same sounds again (Smith, 1978; Costello, 1981–1984).

Instead of repeating the same words over and over again, you need to change not only the words, but the structure as well. In other words, do not simply substitute a couple of words ("Are you going to the river?"); structure carries meaning, too, and the hearing-impaired person's mind as well as her ears will conspire against you to try to confirm the meaning she has already guessed. What you need to do is think of one or two new topic words that you did not use in your original sentence and get her to understand them.

In my case, I might say, "No, *boating.*" If mom still does not get it, I might try, "the river, boating on the river." By then she is probably laughing, saying, "Oh, you mean boating. Were you asking if we were going boating?" Now we are back on track, and I can ask my original question again because I have her looking for the correct meaning behind my words, and not the incorrect meaning she had first created. As much as is possible, we are sharing our personal world views, working on the same topic.

We all have had the mistaken notion that if we repeat things often enough, eventually the meaning will get across. But as you can see, there is a law of diminishing returns. If the hearing-impaired person did not get the meaning after two or three tries, then take the time to stop and think of what you said and what you want to say. Think up a topic word or two describing what you want to say, and try them. Then, when the hearing-impaired person is back on the right track, you can build back up to what you were saying originally.

Doing this may often leave you at a loss for words. You will be tempted to reuse words that were misunderstood the first few times, either because you like them or because you just cannot think of an alternative. My advice here is have patience and practice. You do not need to say something right away, and what you say does not have to be exact. As long as it gets the hearing-impaired person thinking in the right direction, so to speak, you can get her back to your original sentence. And if all else fails, you can spell out the topic word or write it down.

Re-creating Conversation

Improving your communication with a hearing-impaired person actually only involves a couple of easy steps. First, you need to work out a system between yourself and the hearing-impaired person that allows for visual cues to replace subtle or hard to follow conversational cues. Then you need to try to be aware of the hearing-impaired person, so when he or she asks for help, you will notice and answer the question. Second, you may need to become more creative by thinking up new ways to help the hearing-impaired person understand the topic. That means, very simply, you must try to be aware of the needs of those around you, and as much as possible, meet those needs. Sounds simple, doesn't it? Too often it is not.

A great deal of trial and error is involved, and many mistakes are going to be made. Even when you think the system is all set up and running, it will not stop the interruptions or the puzzled looks on the face of the hard of hearing person when he or she has lost the topic or when the conversation circles ("I said boats." "Yes, books." "No, boats." "Books?" "Boats!" "I heard you! Books!"). But creating and using a system will be of vast help. In many ways, communication is a great deal like love: It takes lots of work to keep it alive, but the rewards are infinite.

Twelve

Techniques for Improving Communication

—"Hey! I only see a hard of hearing person once or twice a month!"

—"My hearing-impaired client only visits my office two or three times a year."

—"Every once in a while I deal with a customer who wears a hearing aid, but not very often."

While these statements above may be true now, in all probability, they will not be true for long. As people live longer and our population grows, as more and more people refuse to be turned away or set aside because they happen to suffer from a hearing loss, ever increasing numbers of hearing-impaired people will be entering and staying in the workforce and the marketplace. These people will be our colleagues, our customers, our clients, our patients, our acquaintances, our friends, our family members.

Acquaintances

My mother seems to bring out the best in people. Of course, much of that is because she cares about others and continually pushes her limited hearing to its utmost in an effort to communicate effectively. People seem to respond by pushing themselves and being patient when communicating with her. But it is heartbreaking to see the number of people who turn away from those with hearing problems, turn their backs on them either out of pity or confusion, or from a self-centered reluctance to take the time to try.

What, then, are the consequences of such actions to hearing-impaired people? How long can we expect intelligent, caring, otherwise "normal" individuals to put up with that kind of treatment before they simply give up? Perhaps when one member of a very large club quits, it does not mean very much in the cosmic scheme of things; the club will survive. And perhaps we would feel better if we were not faced with this person's problem any longer, so we would not have to feel guilty or try to figure out what to do about it. But this kind of behavior on our part imperils our community. We lose these peoples' input into the affairs of our lives. We drive them away from participating in the activities of our community and effectively take away their ability to help shape our little corner of the world. Only a very few people have any control over global issues, so most of us concentrate on our towns or cities, clubs or organizations, churches or religious groups to effect change, to mold a better life for us all. People who have a hearing loss have much to contribute, much too much to be pushed aside and made to feel unwelcome because of our failings, our inability to cope with their disability. Theirs is a physical failing, one they are desperately trying to cope with, but one that will never go away, never get better. Ours is an emotional failing, one that will go away, one that is easily overcome with some effort on our part.

The point is that as a person who has only casual contact with someone who is hearing impaired, you only need to remember a couple of things. First, if someone does not respond to a verbal inquiry, it is not necessarily because that person is rude. Look to see if he or she is wearing a hearing aid. Then, stop a moment and try to notice if there is any background noise. Either of these factors can determine whether or not a hearing-impaired person can hear you at all.

Second, take some initiative. Get the person's attention and say hello. If you and the hearing-impaired person are only casual acquaintances, she might not be aware that you would want to talk to her, get to know her better. This is really not much different from dealing with a person who has normal hearing, except that the hearing-impaired person may be a bit more tentative. Remember, she has trouble with communication, and it is harder for her to recognize the signals for beginning a conversation.

As for maintaining the conversation, the hearing-impaired person should clue you in if she needs anything special from you.

After that, all you need to do is remember to face her, not put your back to the light, not cover up your mouth, and speak as carefully as you can.

The Professional

If you are a professional who has regular contact with hard of hearing people, you have not only an emotional stake in good communication, but an economic one as well. The time you take to better understand the needs of this rapidly growing population will pay great dividends in two ways: first, in the professional sense of being able to perform your job or offer your services with greater ease of communication and much less misunderstanding and in the emotional sense of having created understanding; second, a solid client–professional relationship with a person who, under other circumstances, could have felt frustrated, confused, and bewildered. You will be helping hearing-impaired people build confidence in their ability to communicate and solve problems for themselves in professional settings.

The benefits of better communication apply not only to the upper strata of service professionals but to every person who has regular contact with hearing-impaired individuals. My mother's undying loyalty to her favorite grocery store comes as much from the care and effort of each of the store employees as it does from it being close to her home. Another store is about the same distance away, and the items sold there are usually less expensive than in her favorite store, but at her store the checkers have taken the time and cared enough to remember that she is hearing impaired and they look directly at her. They do not ignore her or pretend she is not there so they do not have to take that extra minute to communicate with her. They let her know she is valued. Everyone from the store manager to the box-boys and girls have a smile or a kind word for her. To my way of thinking, these kind and caring people have as much right to the title *professional* as the doctors and tax accountants in the community.

The key here is the word *community*. Community and communication share the same root word. Each defines the interaction between people who live and work together to form a stable group for the mutual benefit of all. Yet, it is so easy not to take that extra step to make sure that all the people of a community feel valued. This is especially true when someone is unable to communicate because this strikes at the very root of the person's ability to function as a group member.

If you are meeting your hearing-impaired client in an office, consider the available lighting and the general acoustics of your office. You might want to move to a conference room or arrange two chairs on the outside of your desk and sit there, facing the client and the best available light source. This dramatically cuts down the distance between you and your client. Office desks can be as much as four feet across, and once you allow for leg room, you may have put as much as six feet between yourself and your client. That may be too much distance for effective communication to take place.

Many professionals greet their clients in the reception area, then escort them to their offices. This is terrific, since a hard of hearing person will have trouble understanding a secretary saying, "Down the hall, turn left, third door on the right," when there are telephones ringing, people talking, and typewriters or printers chugging away.

Beyond that, the key is to use some common sense, try to speak carefully, and be ready to write down any terms your client may not understand.

Health care professionals are in a class by themselves. The intimate, long-term relationships we build with doctors, dentists, nurse practitioners, and others in this industry are different and often deeper than those we build elsewhere in our community. Eve explored this relationship very thoroughly in chapter 5, giving excellent examples of health care professionals who were good, and some who were not so good, communicators. Therefore, I will only add this: Odds are, if you live long enough, you will experience some degree of hearing loss. And at some point in a lifetime, every doctor needs a doctor.

Friends

My mother and I felt that her friends would be the best people to tell you about what friends of hearing-impaired people need to be aware of, or what they need to do in order to keep in touch with

their hearing-impaired friends. Mom wrote to three of her friends
and asked them to respond to any or all of the following questions:

1. What are the hardest things for you to do/remember when
   communicating with a hearing-impaired person?
2. What special things do you do to keep in touch with a
   hearing-impaired person like me?
3. How do you see all this as modifying or changing the
   friendship?
4. How do you perceive me as having changed?

Here is what each of them had to say.

Geranna Fleming: My first conversation with Eve Nickerson
was on the telephone, around 1978. I was a fledgling secretary
in the office of Eve and Bill's long-time attorney. When I offered to have the attorney call her back, she declined, explaining she was hard of hearing and couldn't hear the phone ring.
I didn't quite believe her, as she spoke beautifully and seemed
to respond appropriately to everything I said.

Eve and I really met, though, over the back fence. In 1979 I
had the remarkable luck to move next door to Eve and Bill,
with just an elbow-high, see-through fence between their
backyard (glorious with flowers, green lawn, and artfully sub-
dued shrubs) and my patio. That twelve-foot span, interrupted
only by one forsythia, became our private forum. Leaning into
the fence, we took on levels of conversation that constantly
surprised us both. Perhaps we didn't solve the world's problems, but I know many of mine were more comprehensible
and far less terrifying afterward.

Only gradually did I realize how great Eve's hearing impairment was. Now I know she exploited the brilliant daylight, the
uncommon quiet, and our wonderful sense of comradeship to
capture the shapes and colors of my words, and inveigled me
to rephrase or reorganize a thought she missed the first time.
After the continued marked decline in her hearing these past
several years, she is still the best listener I have ever known,
and I find myself becoming a better listener when in her
presence. The intensity of her concentration is infectious. To
this day I marvel at the energy, resources, and creativity she
gives to the process of communicating with people. I would
find the task both overwhelming and exhausting.

I "work harder" at conversing with Eve as a means of empathizing with the efforts I see her making. This is why I have at least some small glimmer of the enormous energy she puts into what to most of us is a natural and relatively easy aspect of life—verbal communication with those most dear to us. I do regret being unable to call on the phone for a chat, as our schedules don't always allow for frequent personal visits, and I don't live just over that back fence any more. What I do instead is write—usually just a note or short letter—as a means of checking in and checking up. Eve helps me do this because she always writes back.

Eve is one of the most thoughtful, interesting, generous, and intuitively honest people I know. Her impairment did not create any of these qualities. More importantly, she has not permitted her impairment to take any of them away.

Terri Lutze: I'm afraid, each time, that you [Eve] won't understand what I'm saying. I wonder what I'm going to do if the day comes that you won't be able to understand me. Where will our friendship go at that point? What will I have to do to keep our friendship? Will I learn sign language?

When I'm talking with you, I make sure we have eye contact. I speak slowly and carefully. Sometimes I speak so slowly that I forget what I'm trying to say!

When Bill and I are talking with each other, I'm afraid you won't understand or will feel left out. I'm worried that you're not feeling a part of our conversation.

You've changed. You're willing to say, "I'm just human," to talk about your own difficulties, instead of just listening to mine. Partly that's also a change in our friendship, too. It's not just me sharing my feelings and problems; you're sharing yours, too, and it balances.

It must be hard for you to say, "I can't understand. Please repeat that." But it makes me love you more, that you're willing to say, "I don't understand." That's part of friendship: to be honest.

You're asking for your *needs*, not your *wants*. You've separated those two things out. You're not asking to be the center of attention. You've defined the things you *need* to keep a relationship. I'm glad to fill those needs.

Elizabeth Hirsch:

1. What are the hardest things you do or have to remember when communicating with Eve?

Nothing is really hard any more, largely due to her valiant efforts to understand. We have found a quiet, well-lighted place for our conversations. We have accepted the fact that we can no longer *do* things together and converse, so we engage in one *or* the other.

I used to think I had to talk more loudly, which was hard for me because I have a weak, badly projected voice, but Eve has persuaded me that enunciation is far more important than volume. I never trim my vocabulary or subject matter or style of speech. We exchange so well on all topics that it's incredible to me that she is scarcely hearing me at all.

2. What special things do you do to keep in touch with a hearing-impaired person?

Have a regular meeting time to be alone together, for concentrated communication, in a quiet place. Face the person and speak slowly and distinctly. (I don't try to sew or peel apples while I'm talking with Eve.) In a group, try to clue the person in to the subject being discussed.

3. How do you see all this as modifying or changing the friendship?

It has modified our behavior, not our friendship. We can't do the things we used to do together, but the affection, the understanding, the mutual concern have only deepened. I can imagine that if Eve were a lesser person, this might not have been so. But she is a very special person, and knowing someone of her mentality, heart, and spirit is a privilege.

4. How do you perceive Eve as having changed?

I know Eve has been—*is*—frightened. She's afraid of total hearing loss, of losing touch with people; and because of her husband's prolonged illness, afraid of being left alone. She carries a great emotional burden with unsurpassed courage. Her determination to remain cheerful and upbeat sometimes seems a little desperate and her ready laughter is not far removed from tears. But her interests, her actions, smart appearance and even her mode of talking are unaltered. Here is a bright, brave lady caught up in true tragedy not of her own making. If anything positive can be made of such a situation, she will do it. I think this book may be it.

The Family

Truth is neither easy nor kind. It is a knife that slices through our carefully constructed, nicely organized, familiar worlds. It cuts with little regard to politeness or kindness, suitability or convenience. It severs the threads of our lives, often leaving ragged edges dangling forlornly, haphazardly.

And yet truth is at the very core of the journey we, Eve and I, now ask you to make. It will not be an easy journey; it was not easy for us either to make it or to write about it. In this section I am taking off my "party dress," setting aside my pretty phrases, and writing as honestly and straightforwardly as I can about living with a hard of hearing person. Truth may not be comfortable, but I have no greater, more precious gift to give those of you who are struggling to maintain a loving relationship with a hearing-impaired person.

The Three Sins

We are all guilty, at one time or another, of three sins—self-centeredness, pity, and confusion.

There are days when I am tired and irritable, and I just cannot muster up the will to do better for Eve. I am ashamed of these self-centered feelings and I try to do better, but they are there. I guess the only thing we can do about our self-centered reluctance, whatever guise it takes (others are waiting for my services, I have to get some errands done, I have a headache), is to try to recognize it for what it is and be truthful, both to ourselves and to the hard of hearing people in our lives. After all, they do not expect us to have deep, meaningful conversations with them every time they see us. They might not be in the mood or have the time, either. As with your hearing friends, a smile and "Hello, how's it going?" is all that is needed. And if you are in a hurry, say what you would say to a hearing member of the family: "I'd love to chat but I'm running late and really have to go."

As far as I can see, the sin of self-centeredness can be overcome by a dose of plain old-fashioned good manners.

Pity is a harder problem to control. It is often all mixed up in our fears and anxieties for ourselves, our children, or family. After all, if hearing loss can happen to one of them, it could happen to us, and we certainly do not enjoy being reminded of that. I think that the best we can do is try to turn pity around to an awareness of the hearing-impaired person's difficulties.

If we try to be aware of another's problems and creatively attempt to overcome them, to do what we can to minimize them, then we won't have time for reflection, and pity thrives on reflection. It is one of those emotions we seem to have to think about to kick into gear. Try not to give yourself the time. Work at communicating rather than reflecting. Work at getting closer to the person, rather than farther away. Believe me, it is work, but it is one of the most rewarding kinds of work.

Just what does this work consist of? Well, that takes us into the third sin: confusion. At the root of confusion is a lack of understanding of exactly what we are supposed to do. We know that the person cannot hear us very well, and sometimes it seems as though, through no fault of our own, he or she cannot hear us at all. We are not sure what to do or when to do it.

Is it better to ignore a hard of hearing person than take the chance of offending him or her? Are you tired of a hearing-impaired person giving you directions on how to talk (especially if that person is your parent, from whom you have received quite enough instruction)? Are you confused about hearing loss in general, and what your responsibilities to a hearing-impaired person are? Well, I have been. That is really how this book got started. By reading this book, you are taking the first major step in overcoming your confusion—you are learning what you can do about communicating with a hearing-impaired person more effectively.

As far as what to do in everyday situations, the solution is really not very different from the way we should treat all our friends and family members: listen, watch, and try to communicate deliberately and lovingly.

The Truth as I Know It

I would like to talk to you about a few things that I have had to learn the hard way. I noticed early on that my mom heard better on some days than on others, and even in some moments better than other moments. At 6:00 p.m. she would overhear a conversation at the other end of the room, and at 6:30 p.m. she would not understand someone talking to her face to face. All of the other factors were equal—same room, same speaker, same conditions, but she could hardly hear a thing. I began to think that she only heard when or what she wanted to hear. And although I hate to admit it, I once thought that maybe it was psychological. I dismissed the notion right away, but I thought it.

I was wrong. I was wrong to belittle the problems faced by hearing-impaired people, and I was wrong to malign my mother, even in my thoughts.

When we tire, our minds start to deal with information differently than when we are fresh. The mind becomes more impatient, more easily confused, and this is often evidenced in what we term a short attention span. This is a physical reaction to fatigue that researchers are beginning to explore and understand better. The mechanics of moving information through the brain are complex and not thoroughly understood, but we do know that fatigue plays a major role in the mind's ability to comprehend and retain information.

Emotional changes, tiredness, and depression all play important roles in a hearing-impaired person's ability to understand communication. Communicating is very hard work for hearing-impaired people. We hearing people can carry on a conversation with half a mind, but hearing-impaired people must concentrate fully on every nuance and rhythm and sound in order to extract and reconstruct a speaker's meaning. This is high level concentration, and it cannot be kept up indefinitely. My mother, who has worked and trained at this since 1985, has a top concentration time of about four hours. That is four hours out of an eighteen-hour day. Granted, she is severely hard of hearing, so the amount of energy she focuses on keeping up with a conversation is perhaps more than others might need to expend. But she has been trained.

Most people have not had the training necessary to extend their concentration time and thereby extend the time they can expend in understanding conversation. Naturally, they tire quickly, and as they tire, their concentration slips. The end result is that they are not able to track or keep up with the conversation. In other words, they just do not seem to hear as well as they did earlier in the day.

Please understand that this is not because they do not want to hear. Believe me, if there were any way they could, they would. Any degree or type of hearing impairment is terribly confining and isolating, and most people would do anything they could to regain their hearing. But there are genuine medical and physical reasons why a hard of hearing person hears better on some days than on others. The best thing that you can do is to recognize when your spouse or family member is having a bad time of it. At those times, try to keep the conversation to a minimum. If you want to have a nice, long chat, reschedule it for another time. But please do not get discouraged.

Hearing Loss vs. Communication Problems

For a long time I labored under a large misconception. I believed that my mother's hearing impairment was the sole source of her communication problems. Mom set me straight on this. She, like most people in the world who are hearing impaired, has two types of communication problems.

The first is that she misses the words that are spoken to her. The second consists of all the communication problems she brought with her, that were in place before she started to lose her hearing. She talks about these problems extensively in chapters 5 and 6, from her point of view, so I will be brief and talk about them from the communication point of view.

None of us is a perfect communicator. We all have faults that lead us to say inappropriate things or to act in ways we regret. Perhaps we do not listen as well as we should. Perhaps we are too talkative or too quiet, too hasty or too slow. Perhaps we have begun to take the people we love for granted. Whatever our communication faults, a hearing impairment will have a tendency to magnify them and perhaps, for the first time, bring them into the forefront of a relationship.

For years these problems may have been manageable. They were probably little problems that the members of a close relationship could ignore or learned to work around. But the onset of a hearing impairment in an already established relationship can force these problems into the open, creating havoc in the relationship.

Comments such as the following are often heard among couples when one partner has a hearing loss.

—"He tells me, 'Yes, I heard you,' but then he gets mad at me a day later because he says I never told him."

—"She only wears her hearing aid when she wants to listen to the television, not to me."

—"When I ask him to repeat something, he shouts at me and hurts my feelings."

—"He ignores me when he comes home from work, as if he can't be bothered to listen to what I have to say."

—"She doesn't ask me about what's happened to me during the day any more."

Many couples say that they didn't have these kinds of problems before the hearing loss began. We can blame a hearing impairment all we want to, but the truth is that many communication problems do not start with a hearing loss. By all means, the couple should go to an audiologist or hearing aid dealer to check out the newest hearing aids and assistive devices. But be aware that a new hearing aid will only help solve the first type of communication problems. If there seems to be more to the problem than missing words and you cannot find solutions between you, please consider seeing a counselor or therapist together or separately. Many professionals are trained to help people with the second type of communication problems. Many major universities and most cities and counties have staff counselors to help people in just this situation. Many services are free or have sliding fee schedules, so cost should not deter you. If you cannot solve your communication problems by yourselves, if you feel that your problems go beyond missing words and you are having trouble getting them straightened out, then please, *please*, get help.

Never Mind . . .

If I have one overriding piece of advice for the family of a hearing-impaired person, it is this: Never say, "never mind."

It is not all right for Eve to miss what I say to her. She tries very hard not to interrupt, but if I make a comment to her that she misses and asks me to repeat, and I say, "never mind," it is as if I slapped her in the face. Just what is she supposed to think? That I didn't want to talk to her, to convey information? That I didn't want her to feel included? That what I had to say is suddenly unimportant? That I changed my mind? That her hearing impairment is a nuisance to me? That she is bothering me or putting me out?

Sometimes she asks me to repeat someone else's remark, a remark that I thought was trivial or completely unimportant. But it is not for me to judge what is or is not worthy to pass on to her. If she asks me to repeat something, to relay a comment to her, I do it. Anything less is treating her as if she were stupid, as if her wants and needs were unreasonable. I must do her the honor of respecting her intelligence.

She hears many comments differently than I do. It could be that she thought she heard something that startled or alarmed her. By honestly relating the comment, even if it was a silly piece of nonsense, I could very well be setting her mind at ease, helping her separate out what she thought she heard from what was really said.

Perhaps the comment was embarrassing, a comment that I would be uncomfortable repeating right then. In that case, I can say, "Later," and mean it. There are always moments in any gathering, no matter how formal or informal, when I can seek her out, take her aside, and tell her what was said. She isn't asking me to comment on it, to judge the speaker. I just tell her what I remember the speaker saying. If repeating the unkind comment would embarrass me or make me feel uncomfortable, I just say, clearly and without apology, "What that person said wasn't kind, and I don't want to repeat it to *anyone.*" She will certainly understand my position.

But please, if you love or have affection for a person who misses words, never say, "never mind."

Having The Answer

Since my mother and I began writing this book, we cannot tell you how many times we have been told, "My father/mother/ brother/sister/cousin has a hearing aid, but won't wear it," or "My father/mother/brother/sister/cousin needs a hearing aid but won't go get one." Then the person who has made this statement waits for us to impart The Answer to the big question: How do I convince my father/mother/brother/sister/cousin to purchase and/or wear a hearing aid?

If that's the question, we don't have The Answer. Part of the reason is that every person is different. There are many types of hearing loss and hearing aids, and there are a hundred reasons why a person might not want to wear a hearing aid. The real answer is at once much more complex, and much more simple. Finding your answer will start you on your own journey, one that will stretch your mind and your heart. For us, it started with this premise: It is very difficult for a person with normal hearing to truly comprehend what hearing-impaired people go through.

You have already taken the first step by reading this book, cover to cover. You have begun to understand the problems a hearing-impaired person faces—real, physical problems, some of which can never fully be overcome. Also, you can visit your local libraries, and check out books and read the journals of hearing loss support organizations. If you are lucky enough to live close to a college or university, try their libraries, too.

You can learn firsthand by creating opportunities for hearing-impaired people to explain their difficulties, explain what they are hearing, how difficult it is to adjust to some sounds, and where the trouble spots are. Then listen to what they tell you; really listen. Who knows? You just might come up with some pretty creative solutions to some of the problems they are experiencing.

However, gaining understanding is only half the battle, and the easy half at that. The other half is putting the knowledge you gain to good use, and that's the tough part. You can lecture until the cows come home, but if the hearing-impaired person's reluctance is based on fear then all the academic, logical arguments in the world won't mean a thing.

I found, time and time again, that the best thing I could do was forget about linguistics, acoustics, hearing aids, and medicine and tell my mom, in words and deeds, "I love you. I love you even though you cannot hear all of my words. I will love you even if you never hear another sound. And no matter what, I will not give up on you or on communicating with you."

If there is an Answer, maybe that's it. At least it is as close as I have ever come.

I have found that conversations with my mother now are very different from the conversations I had with her when she could hear better. Instead of going forward, bounding from topic to topic, moving always quickly and surely in any direction that took our fancy, our conversations are rather spiral. We start talking, back up and revise, check meanings and intentions, then move forward again. It is very deliberate, very careful communication. In many ways we work much harder at helping each other by sitting in a special place, talking in a certain way, and watching each other. I never really watched people before when I talked to them, never used to look at them and see them. With Mom, I have to. I can tell by looking at her face whether or not she has understood what I have said, and she watches me to gather all the visual cues she can.

I guess what I am trying to say is that even though you do everything you can to make communication with your hearing-impaired friend or family member better, it will never be the way it was. But if you work hard, if you are patient and diligent, the dialogue will be just as rich, just as fulfilling as it was before. There is communication after hearing loss. There can be love and growth in the silent places. You can make it so.

Afterword

In the six years I have had a cochlear implant, the external paraphernalia of my implant have become increasingly user friendly. My transmitter (the size of a quarter, but very light) is easily and gently held by magnets to the receiver, which is embedded under my scalp in the bone behind my ear. I forget it is there most of the time. The microphone, which hangs over my ear, is smaller than most behind-the-ear hearing aids. The two-strand wire that connects these to my speech processor is thin and flexible, and it easily tucks into clothing. The speech processor (I have the latest model, called a Miniprocessor) is encased in smooth, gray plastic. It measures $2^{5}/_{8}"$ by $3^{1}/_{2}"$ by $^{3}/_{4}"$—small enough and light enough to fit into a shirt pocket or, in my case, into one of the soft cloth pouches I make and sew into bras.

Obviously, such complex electronics cannot be allowed to get wet or be hit or crushed. I cannot wear them when I bathe, sleep, play in the water, or participate in sports that involve body contact. That doesn't stop me from using hand signals to swim, sail, play basketball, soccer, or any other sport.

The processor is expensive ($5,000). Mine came with a three-year warranty, and when the warranty expires, I can buy insurance from the manufacturer. This is a new technology and I go to great lengths to protect my precious lifelines. One implant user I know operates heavy machinery in the forests of Alaska. He had a friend design and build a special leather holster for his processor. He says he would not dream of operating his potentially dangerous machinery without the safety factor provided by his implant.

Whenever I leave home, I carry extra AA-sized batteries. I use high grade, rechargeable ones, one at a time, and each one lasts about ten hours before I need to recharge it. Extra batteries and the recharger go with me when I travel.

When I first began to wear my equipment (three weeks after surgery), I continuously returned to my audiologist to have my personal program or "map" adjusted, or even changed completely, seeking optimum input. This required that I explain exactly what I was perceiving—what felt good and what was troubling—in order to improve the program.

I experienced some anxiety and stress during the early stages. I was fearful that I would not easily interpret speech, that I would not function at all well with this new technology. At the same time, I felt enormous determination to improve and gratitude for the chance to stay connected to the world. At the end of a year of working with the implant, I was elated with the improvement.

One of the adjustments I had to make was to learn to change the dial settings on my processor more frequently than I would on a hearing aid. Overwhelming, sometimes hurtful, input results when someone close to me turns on a machine or rustles a newspaper; when I move out into noisy automobile traffic; and when I turn on a kitchen fan, a microwave oven, or even a typewriter. Now my hand moves quickly to the dials. I soon grew so used to the implant that I could change the settings without looking at them. People who don't know me often give me strange looks when I reach into my bra to adjust the dials; but that's all right. I explain and we all get a good laugh.

It is difficult to explain what this mysterious input feels like, this electrical stimulation to the auditory nerve that tries to simulate real sound. But, I'll try.

There are probably as many explanations as there are those of us who wear cochlear implants. Most of us have needed many months, sometimes years, to relearn the world of sound. Many of us describe human voices as resembling a mixture of Donald Duck and Woody Woodpecker; in other words, voices sound scratchy and lack the richness of voice tones and pitch. To make matters worse, we lose intelligibility when more than five feet away from the speaker.

We often feel we are receiving too little useful information, even when we turn the volume to high. But more is not always better; we learn to turn the volume down against background noise to catch what we can. We are always experimenting. We strain to understand, wish for more information from mushy speech sounds, and yearn for others to pronounce more precisely and slowly. Yet those priceless moments do occur when all our needs are met, and for a while we converse with such ease that we forget we cannot hear.

Some implant wearers say they can use the telephone for work and socializing, others say they can use it in a limited fashion, and still others say they cannot use it at all except with telephone/ typewriter devices and relay systems.

Music, for me, is real only when I sing out loud to myself. All I can perceive from external sources is the rhythm and a few scratchy, discordant sounds. Others say they have slowly retrained themselves and gradually appreciate music again.

The sounds of our environment take time to re-identify, then remember, then recognize. Some unexpected noise sources remain forever a mystery. Slowly, over months, the sounds of our daily lives begin to make sense again.

This has been, for me, a difficult process. When Dr. F. Owen Black tried to surgically insert the wire with twenty-two electrodes into my inner ear, his efforts were blocked by bone growth in my cochlea. Only great skill and patience on his part gave me the gift of eleven usable electrodes. One would therefore guess that I do only half as well as patients who utilize all twenty-two electrodes. Yet doctors and audiologists who work with implant patients say this isn't true. Some patients who would seem to have everything in their favor do not do well. Others with even fewer than eleven electrodes function well to a limited extent.

The professionals who work with implant patients tell me that there is no way of predicting ahead of time who will be more successful. We all know what helps: strong support from family and friends, a determination to succeed, a realistic understanding of the limitations and the hard work, and the knowledge that discouragement must always be overcome.

I grow impatient with the lack of input and the static-like distortion that my brain strives to interpret. But take away my devices and I am in a panic. With them on I relax, filled with joy that I can still perceive so much and understand so many of those missing words.

Eve Nickerson

Part Four

Resources

Resources

Organizations

SHHH: Self Help for Hard of Hearing People

Self Help for Hard of Hearing People, Inc. (SHHH) is a volunteer, international organization of hard of hearing people, their relatives, and friends. SHHH is devoted to the welfare and interests of those who cannot hear well. There are more than 225 SHHH support groups in the United States, and these groups are a great source of information, help, and encouragement.

SHHH publishes a journal about hearing loss and coping techniques six times a year (a subscription is included in the modest national membership dues). This is a truly helpful publication that covers a huge number of topics, including new hearing aids and electronic devices available on the market, book reviews, and "how to" and advice columns. In every issue we learn something or gain greater insights. The *SHHH* journal is a wonderful resource.

For more information about SHHH, their publications or support groups, please contact:

SHHH
7800 Wisconsin Avenue
Bethesda, MD 20814
(301) 657-2248 (Voice)
(301) 657-2249 (TT*)

Note: In this section we will use TT to refer to any telephone device (TTY, TDD, or TT) that allows deaf and hard of hearing people to use a telephone.

American Tinnitus Association

The American Tinnitus Association (ATA) is a nonprofit corporation dedicated to helping tinnitus patients and to supporting tinnitus research. The ATA provides information about tinnitus, health professionals who treat tinnitus, self-help groups and the problems of stress, as well as some practical, down-to-earth solutions for eliminating stress. This information is well worth having, even if you do not have tinnitus. If you are experiencing feedback or noise interference with your hearing aids, you may well be experiencing the stress that goes along with listening to such noise. The American Tinnitus Association pamphlet "Coping with the Stress of Tinnitus" can give you valuable, useful information.

The American Tinnitus Association also has a quarterly newsletter to which you can subscribe. The newsletter contains up-to-date information on all the newest advances in fighting or coping with tinnitus.

To request a copy of ATA's pamphlets, enclose a self-addressed, stamped (2 oz., first class) business envelope (#10 or larger). Two of their most popular pamphlets are "Information About Tinnitus" and "Coping with the Stress of Tinnitus." If you are interested in becoming a member of ATA, write to them at the following address:

The American Tinnitus Association
P.O. Box 5
Portland, OR 97207
(503) 248-9985 (Voice)

Other Organizations

In addition to the few we have highlighted, there are many, many organizations across the country, all doing wonderful things. Each organization focuses on a slightly different group of people with slightly different needs. It may be well worth your time to contact some that seem to best suit your needs and find out more about them.

Association of Late-Deafened Adults
P.O. Box 641763
Chicago, IL 60664-1763
(312) 604-4192 (TT)
Resource and information center; publishes *ALDA News*

Better Hearing Institute
5021-B Backlick Road
Annandale, VA 22003
(703) 642-0580 (Voice)
Information, resources, and doctor referrals; publishes *The Communicator*

IBM National Support Center for Persons with Disabilities
P.O. Box 2150
Atlanta, GA 30055
Information about how computers (and other technology) can assist people with hearing loss or other handicaps at home, in school, and at work

American Speech-Language-Hearing Association
National Association for Hearing and Speech Action
10801 Rockville Pike
Rockville, MD 20852
(301) 897-5700 (Voice/TT)
(800) 638-8255 (Voice, Helpline)
Services and information on communication disorders

National Hearing Aid Society
20361 Middlebelt Road
Livonia, MI 48152
(313) 478-2610 (Voice)
(800) 521-5247 (Voice, Hearing Aid Helpline)
Consumer information and referral services

National Information Center on Deafness
Gallaudet University
800 Florida Avenue NE
Washington, DC 20002
(202) 651-5051 (Voice)
(202) 651-5052 (TT)
Information on hearing loss, deafness, and Gallaudet University

Telecommunications for the Deaf, Inc.
8719 Colesville Road, Suite 300
Silver Spring, MD 20910-3919
(301) 589-3786 (Voice)
(301) 589-3006 (TT)
Special-interest organization supporting technology for deaf and hard of hearing people; sells equipment directly to consumers

Videotapes

"Read My Lips" Speechreading Tapes

The "Read My Lips" videotapes offer a complete speechreading course. The tapes are excellent, beautifully produced, and extremely helpful for people who wish to begin learning speechreading. They are also helpful for those who would like to sharpen their skills. There are six tapes in the series, each one a complete set of lessons in itself. This means that you do not have to send for all six. You can get them one at a time and spend as much time with each one as you like before you move on. Because the lessons are on videotape, you can go at your own pace, repeat as often as you like, and study at times that are convenient for you. Any spoken words are captioned, so you can work alone.

We are very excited about these tapes. Eve was so impressed with how wonderfully clear the lessons were and how much she learned from the first tape, that she has sent for the second. If you want to find out more about the tapes, you can write or call for a brochure describing the tapes and information on how to order them.

"Read My Lips" Speechreading Tapes
Speechreading Laboratory, Inc.
P.O. Box 941
Mustang, OK 73064
(800) 433-6370

Support Electronics

With the advent of the microchip, the support electronics industry has boomed. Many devices exist today that simply were not available ten years ago, and more are finding their way into the market every day. Belonging to a support group or several organizations can keep you in touch with new products as they become available. What follows is a brief list of a few of the personal support electronics on today's market and how you can find out more about them.

TT/TTY/TDD

The name of this device has changed over the years. TTY stands for teletypewriter, or teletype for short. Before personal computers and modems allowed us to send and receive a conversation in written format, teletype machines were used. Basically, they are typewriters that allow two people to type to each other via telephone lines. Probably the most easily recognizable teletype system belongs to Western Union. These machines are very large and bulky, and for personal use have been replaced by the TDD or TT.

TDD stands for telecommunications device for the deaf. This is the term currently used for these nifty machines. They are small (about the size of a portable typewriter or laptop computer) and hook into a standard electrical outlet. They perform the same function as a TTY: two people who each have a telephone and a TDD can type back and forth to each other.

The problem with the name TDD is that it infers that this machine is only for people who are deaf. But the TDD has wider applications. People who have speech disorders can use TDDs as well. That is why the new name, TT for text telephone, is catching on.

TTs are manufactured by many different companies and come in many models. Some come with a memory so that conversations can be stored, and some come with printers. TTs can be read in two ways: the characters appear on a small screen and move across the screen, or the message is printed out as the other person types it. Some machines are capable of doing both.

There are advantages and disadvantages to both systems. It can be very helpful to have a printed record of the conversation in progress, but printers mean print heads and ribbons and loading paper, which can be a hassle and provide more things to go wrong. Another consideration might be portability. Some TTs hook directly into the phone line (direct connect), eliminating the need for a telephone. Most TTs, though, have a cradle for the handset of a telephone that is connected to the phone line. If you use different phones (because you are traveling or taking the TT to work every day), then you will probably also need to purchase handset adapters so the handsets will fit correctly into the cradle. Some telephones (the flat phone handsets that don't have the big round ends) may not work in the TT cradle. This is when having a direct connect TT would be a distinct advantage.

Our advice is to research carefully, look at many different models and styles, read the available literature, and then make a careful, reasoned decision based on your needs.

TT Modem

A modem is an electronic translation device that allows computer signals to be sent over phone lines to another computer. A TT modem turns a home computer into a TT device.

Visual Signaling Devices

Signaling devices use adapters to flash a light or turn on a fan when the phone, doorbell, or fire alarm rings. The adapter is a small box that usually has a phone or electrical connection cord and a power cord. The phone cord hooks into one side of a split phone jack (a phone jack that has been doubled with a small device) while the regular phone jack is in the other side. The power plug simply plugs into an outlet. The box also has another power outlet for the signal light or fan. There are many uses for this gadget, and different models are available to accommodate those uses.

Closed Caption Decoder or Telecaption Decoder

More and more programming on TV is being closed captioned, including many daytime serials, the evening news programs, regular nighttime programming, and sports programs.

The symbol adopted by the industry for marking those programs or rental movies that are closed captioned looks like a television screen with one slanted leg. If a program is closed captioned, you can see this symbol (or just the letters "CC") in weekly and daily television listings (usually at the end of the description of the program or right after the name of the program).

The closed captioned symbol also appears on videocassette rental movies. Sometimes it is on the back, next to the running time, sometimes it is on the front, in the bottom left hand corner. It is also on the label of the actual tape box. It pays to check, because some movies are taped with and without closed captions. Your video rental store clerks can help you find the movies that are closed captioned.

Eve particularly adores captioned movies because it means she can enjoy movies again (one of the things she really missed). Not all rental release movies are closed captioned, but many are. If you are or become a fan of captioned rental movies or television programs, please write the studios or the distributors or television stations and tell them so. We need to encourage the industries to continue and expand the practice.

Watching a closed captioned program is just like watching a subtitled foreign film. The words that the people are saying flash across the top or the bottom of the screen. When the decoder is turned off, the program will look like it normally does, but when it is turned on, the captions appear.

Captions are a little bothersome at first for a person with normal hearing. I tended to read the captions, even though I could hear the actors perfectly well. But I soon learned to ignore the captions, and Bill, my father, says he does not really even notice them any more. When you consider how wonderful it is for someone who is hard of hearing to be able to understand the nightly network news or favorite programs and movies, it is well worth it.

Some TV manufacturers build the closed caption decoder into the TV. All TV sets with screens 13 inches or larger manufactured in the U.S. after July 1, 1993, must have built-in decoders (see ADA, this section). That's good news because hooking up a closed caption decoder can be confusing. Connecting the decoder to a television is fairly straightforward, but hooking it up with both a TV and a VCR is a more complicated job. Don't hesitate to contact an expert or, at least, someone who has done it before.

You may experience a signal loss (slightly blurred or fuzzy picture) if the signal is being run through both the closed caption decoder and the VCR. These are both excellent things to consider before buying a closed caption decoder. If your TV is fairly old and you were thinking of buying a new one soon anyway, you might want to purchase a new TV that has the decoder built in rather than buy the decoder now and a TV next year.

Neither of these reasons was good enough for Eve and Bill to consider waiting. The closed caption decoder has brought Eve hours and hours of entertainment, information, and family fun. If it meant I had to hook the darned thing up for her once a week, I'd do it. And the slightly blurry picture is a small price to pay for her enjoyment.

Timer on a Rope

Not all useful electronics are state-of-the-art gadgets found in catalogues or fancy device stores. In fact, some of the most used and useful items can be found in the most unlikely places, such as kitchen supply stores.

About five years ago I gave Eve a small, wind-up kitchen timer as a Christmas present. She carried that thing all over the house with her. No longer able to hear the timer on the kitchen stove, this was the only way she could know when something she was cooking or baking was done without spending the whole time watching the clock or sitting in the kitchen.

Alas, the timer broke one October day, so off I went to my favorite kitchen supply store to find her another. Lo and behold, what did I find, but a timer on a rope. Well, that was *that* year's Christmas present, and it was twice as successful as the original timer. This timer is almost foolproof. She cannot put it down and forget it because it is hanging around her neck. She uses it constantly for everything from baking cookies to changing the lawn sprinkler. She does not even have to worry if she has her hearing aids on or off when the timer rings. She can feel the vibration because the timer is resting against her chest.

I recently went back to the kitchen supply store to see if they still carried the timer on a rope, and I am sorry to say they did not. But they did have a timer on a clip that one could either clip to a shirt or pants pocket or turn into a timer on a rope by slipping a heavy piece of string or cord through it.

I was reminded once again that a little creative thinking and imagination can make as big a difference in someone's life as the most expensive electronic wonder. There are resources all around us if we are willing to look.

Sources of Information

Tele-Consumer Hotline

This hotline, founded by the Telecommunications Research and Action Center and the Consumer Federation of America, is a great source of information. Upon request they will send you the "Shoppers' Guide for Telephone Users with Special Needs" packet, which includes information about products, their prices, and where you can purchase them. I found it particularly useful in helping me decide which TT I wanted to buy.

Tele-Consumer Hotline
1910 K Street, NW, Suite 610
Washington, DC 20006
1-800-332-1124 (Voice/TT)
(202-223-4371 inside Washington, DC)

AT&T

AT&T carries useful, well made electronic devices for hard of hearing people. Since AT&T has its own research facilities, they often have the most up-to-date electronics on the market. Not only that, they are prompt about sending you their catalogue full of products.

If you are beginning to have trouble with telephones or the television, or just want to know about some of the products available in communication electronics for hearing-impaired people, get their catalogue. They offer a whole range of electronic devices and will gladly send you a catalogue that describes the devices, shows pictures of them, and gives their prices. An order form is included in the booklet.

In the catalogue are listed such useful devices as the "Pocket Talker" and the amplified receiver. An amplified receiver has a dial that increases loudness to any desired level, and it can replace any regular telephone receiver as long as the electronics are compatible. This amplified receiver can be used in conjunction with a hearing aid. If you use an amplified receiver, experiment to find whether you hear better with or without your hearing aid. If you use the amplified receiver with a hearing aid, try moving the receiver around your hearing aid to discover the angle that gives you the best input.

I have talked with the people at both the Special Needs Center and the National Equipment Center for AT&T, and everyone I came in contact with was kind, helpful, and concerned; all in all a great bunch of people, doing a great job. To obtain the special needs equipment catalogue with electronics available for assisting hard of hearing people, contact:

AT&T National Special Needs Center
2110 Route 46, Suite 310
Parsippany, N.J. 07054–1315
1-800-223-1222 (Voice/TT)

SHHH

Self Help for Hard of Hearing People, Inc. sponsors support group meetings. Every so often (once or twice a year) those meetings will be devoted to personal support electronics or assistive listening devices. In Portland there is just such a meeting about every six months. The group invites noted researchers in the field of electronics for hearing-impaired people to come and bring all sorts of devices. Members of the group can try out the devices and talk to the researchers and others who have perhaps used the devices.

For more information, contact SHHH at the address given at the beginning of this section. They can put you in touch with your closest local chapter of SHHH.

The Phone Book

Another place I can't recommend highly enough is your local phone book. Look under *electronics, hearing aids, deaf,* and *associations,* and also look in the reference pages for stores and organizations in your area that can help you discover the world of personal support electronics.

The Ultimate Personal Support "Device"

Lastly, one of the most effective support devices for someone with a hearing loss (especially someone who lives alone) isn't an electronic device at all, it's a dog. Just as seeing eye dogs have been trained to help blind people, hearing ear dogs have been trained to assist people who are hard of hearing or deaf. When a baby cries or a doorbell rings, these dogs are trained to go get their owners and lead them to the source of the noise. To find out more about hearing ear dogs, write to

Canine Companions for Independence
Executive Office
P.O. Box 446
Santa Rosa, CA 95402

Hearing Ear Dog Program
Executive Office
P.O. Box 213
West Boylston, MA 01583

Red Acre Farm Hearing Dog Center
109 Red Acre Road
P.O. Box 278
Stow, MA 01775

Public Support Electronics

Approximately 20,000 public buildings in the United States in-cluding churches and lecture halls, currently have some type of Assistive Listening System (ALS) to make sounds accessible for hard of hearing people, and the list is growing. The technologies they employ vary—audio induction loops; FM, AM, and hard wired systems; infrared systems, etc. SHHH maintains an inven-tory of places with assistive listening systems (PALS) and would be happy to help you locate such places in your hometown.

For more information on how to identify those places in your community that have assistive listening systems, write to SHHH. Please include a self-addressed, stamped (2 ounces, first class), business envelope along with your request for information. You may have to specify certain areas, types of businesses, or specific club or religious affiliations if you live near or in an area that has a very large number of PALS. But the first step is to write to SHHH.

Americans with Disabilities Act (ADA)

In July of 1990, President Bush signed into law the the Ameri-cans with Disabilities Act. Drawing on the Civil Rights Act of 1964 and the Rehabilitation Act of 1973, this law specifically calls for equal treatment for all people regardless of any physical or mental restrictions. The law is sweeping, demanding full and equal use and enjoyment of public accommodations, employment opportunities, public services, public transportation (except aircraft or certain rail operations), and telecommunications.

Although you may not see yourself as disabled, many of the effects of the ADA will touch your life. What follows are some of the features of the act that will have direct impact on hearing-impaired people.

The ADA has already changed the way this country does business, and this is just the beginning. Basically, the law states that it is your right, as a citizen, to hear a council meeting, a state art commission meeting, a zoning meeting. If you are hard of hearing and need special public support electronics or ALSs, then, as far as possible, your needs must be met.

In the area of employment, an employer is required to hire you even if you are hard of hearing, if you are the person best qualified for the job. The employer must also provide any devices necessary for you to function effectively, as long as purchasing them is not an "undue burden." The size of the employer's organization obviously affects the concept of undue burden. You may offer to pick up some of the cost if it is too high. Studies conclude that over 70 percent of the devices cost less than $400 and 50 percent less than $50. Any employee who develops a hearing loss on the job can expect and, indeed, request or demand accommodation.

SHHH is working with the National Center for Law and Deafness to assist hospitals, hotels, and motels in the areas necessary for communication access for hearing-impaired people. The four components they outline in their program are technology, staff training, identification of those in need, and interpreter services. A great deal of improvement in accommodations will result, as well as increased awareness of the needs of a large segment of the population.

Telephones with amplified receivers are already in place in many airports and public buildings where there are five or more phones. They are available upon request in hospitals and many hotel/motel chains. Ask for them ahead of time, if possible. More amplified telephones will be installed as time goes on, especially if requests for them are frequent.

AT&T has designed a "Public Phone 2000" program, offering travelers an array of user-friendly services no other public phone company provides. These include, at one small phone station, a dataport for laptop computers or fax machines, built-in keyboards to access electronic mail, and a 9-inch color monitor displaying graphics and text. The phone is hearing aid compatible, with volume control buttons on the handset. Its keyboard can be used as a TT (text telephone). Initially tested at Newark and Kennedy airports, they will soon be in additional airports (eventually 85), in nine of the ten top hotel chains, and in most major convention centers.

Telecommunications Relay Services (TRS)

TRS is the new name for a service that's been around for a while (dual party relay system, messages relay system, or TDD relay). TRS helps a person with a hearing or speech problem who has a TT to communicate over the telephone system with the help of a communications assistant.

Formerly called a relay operator, a communications assistant (CA) acts as a go-between. If you have a TT, you can dial the relay service and type (or tell by voice) the number and person you wish to reach. The CA will call the person and act as a go-between, listening to one response and typing it for the TT user, and reading the TT response back to the listener. If a hearing person wishes to telephone someone with a TT, the process works the same way only in reverse.

There are other variations on this system, such as voice carryover, where the CA only assists in one side of the conversation. For example, the hearing-impaired person talks directly to the other person, and the CA just listens and waits. Then when the hearing person replies, the CA types the answer for the TT user.

Answering Services

At this point in your life, telephone conversations may or may not be causing you some problems. My mother can get along over the phone in a limited fashion if she knows the topic of the conversation and knows who the caller is. Even so, she has to struggle. She has the most trouble when she answers the phone rather than initiates the call, since she has no idea who is calling or why. This problem has been made worse because of my father's illness; he cannot always comfortably answer the phone. Their solution was to engage an answering service.

My parents have used the same answering service for years. Dad first started with it when he went into business for himself. The exchange that he chose was recommended to him by a business acquaintance as one that gave dependable, excellent service.

Much to my amazement, I found that the answering service was managed by someone I had known in high school, and Jolene and I renewed our friendship. When I returned from California, Jolene gave me a job as an office secretary, and I did secretarial chores for her while I looked for a teaching position. Economics being what they are, I continued with her even after I started teaching, so I was there when she started offering a brand new service to her customers—the message printer.

I took one look at the message printer, thought about Mom and Dad, and said, "Let's give it a try." The problem with a traditional answering service is that one still must pick up messages over the phone. This does not help hearing-impaired people at all. The message printer bridged this gap. It is very small (about 4″ wide, 8″ deep, and 2″ tall), and it plugs into the back of any normal phone. The customer call forwards (a service offered by phone companies in most parts of the country) his or her phone to the answering service, so that any calls coming to the customer are automatically sent to the answering service. When my parents want to pick up their messages, all they have to do is press a button on the message printer and their messages are printed out for them on a little strip of paper.

Mom not only uses the answering service/message printer combination in the way most other people use it (to pick up her messages), she also uses it as a backup whenever she is on the phone. If she makes a call and the phone is already connected to the answering service, she is all set. (When a phone is on call forwarding, it can be still used to call out. Only incoming calls are redirected.) If Mom gets confused or is not able to understand the person she has called, she tells the person to hang up and call her right back. This will connect the caller to the answering service. The caller gives the answering service a message and Mom will push the button that prints out the message and promptly call the person back.

If the phone is not connected to the answering service, Mom tells the caller to hang up and wait two minutes while she connects her phone to the answering service. Then the caller can dial Mom's number, reach the answering service, and give them the message. If necessary, Mom then phones back to the caller, and they can communicate effectively. It sounds complicated, but it really works. Her family and friends are old hands at it, too. She says that just knowing she has that backup system helps her to stay calm and get much more out of phone conversations than she normally could have.

But choosing a good answering service is not easy. It is not just a matter of getting the right equipment. We asked Jolene Corey, the manager of Business Telephone Exchange, Inc. (Portland, Oregon) to address some basic questions about answering services, and this is what she had to say:

1. What are the different types of answering services?

There are three types of answering services—those staffed with live operators using computer technology, including portable message printers; those staffed with live operators without computer assistance; and those using recording devices. Each type of answering service can answer calls and record messages, but for hearing-impaired clients, the ability to retrieve messages on a printer or pager, wherever they may be, is vital. The message printers are small enough to fit easily in an ordinary briefcase and will plug into and retrieve messages from any phone with the proper jack. Pagers will easily fit into a pants or shirt pocket.

2. How does a person go about choosing a good answering service?

A referral is the best way to find a good answering service, but you should also take into consideration the size of the bureau and the average number of accounts per operator. The smaller bureau is usually capable of giving more personalized service, but a larger bureau that allocates fewer accounts per operator can be as good as, if not better than, a smaller bureau that is understaffed.

The personnel at the answering service you choose should be stable. Try to find an answering service with a low turnover rate. If you are constantly dealing with a trainee, your service will not be up to par.

Usually the telephone answering equipment of the bureau is not too important if the answering service is very small, but the equipment at the larger bureau is very important. If one or two operators have to be kept up-to-date any equipment will do, but when many operators need to keep abreast of the activities of hundreds of clients, the assistance of modern technology is vital. With the aid of computers, the bureau can have each client's account updated whenever a client calls in or writes, and this information is automatically brought up on a computer screen whenever the client's phone is answered by any operator. With the hearing-impaired client in mind, computer-assisted equipment is very important because the client can retrieve messages with a portable printer that plugs into a modular phone jack usually found in most homes and offices.

Another way a client can pick up messages is with an Alpha-Pager. This is a pager that has a small screen and displays the typed message. The message can be saved, making this pager very useful for people on the go. They can save the messages they need until they have a chance to write them down or get in touch with the callers. Vibrator and light models are available for clients who are around noisy equipment or are hearing impaired.

3. What can an answering service do for a hearing-impaired client? What can't it do?

Live answering service can provide a vital link between the hearing-impaired person and the outside world, to people who do not have TT (TDD/TTY) machines. The good answering service operator can elicit a more complete message than a recorder and can be on the lookout for a specific person that the hearing-impaired client would like to get a detailed message to or from. The live answering service operator can also call someone for the hearing-impaired person, ask specific questions for him or her, and then relay the answers back via an electronic transmittal to a printer or pager.

4. Based on your experience as a past president of the NorthWest Telephone Answering Service Association, about how much does a good answering service cost per month?

The cost for an answering service, including an electronic message printer, should be between $45 and $65 per month, depending upon the volume of calls. If the customer has a high call volume (for example, if the answering service takes more than fifty calls a month for the client), then the costs will probably be higher.

As you can see, a good answering service with all the equipment and people to help you does not come cheap. But in Eve's case, it costs almost nothing when compared with her being able to deal with emergencies, to make appointments, to stay in touch with her family and friends, and to know she is not helpless when it comes to phone conversations.

If you are interested in looking into an answering service for your business or your home, do your research. Jolene has given you all the information you need to make a start. Write down your questions, go visit the answering services in your area, and tabulate the responses you get. A bad answering service is worse than no answering service at all. But a good one can make your life a whole lot easier.

Bibliography

Abercrombie, David. "Paralanguage." *The British Journal of Disorders of Communication* 3, (1): April 1968 (pp 55–59).

Basso, K. H. " 'To Give Up On Words': Silence in Western Apache Culture." In *Language and Social Context,* edited by Pier Paolo Gigliolo. Middlesex, England: Penguin Books, 1972.

Bennett, Jonathan. *Linguistic Behavior.* Cambridge: Cambridge University Press, 1976.

Bernstein, B. "Social Class, Language and Socialization." In *Language and Social Context,* edited by Pier Paolo Giglioli. Middlesex, England: Penguin Books, 1972.

Birdwhistell, Ray L. *Kinesics and Context: Essays on Body Motion Communication.* Philadelphia: University of Pennsylvania Press, 1970.

Bornstein, Diane D. *An Introduction to Transformational Grammar.* Cambridge, Mass.: Winthrop Publishers, 1977.

Britton, James. *Language and Learning.* Middlesex, England: Penguin Books, 1970.

Brown, Penelope, and Stephen Levinson. "Universals in Language Usage: Politeness Phenomena." In *Questions and Politeness: Strategies in Social Interaction,* edited by Ester N. Goody. London: Cambridge University Press, 1978.

Campbell, Jeremy. *Grammatical Man: Information, Entropy, Language, and Life.* New York: Simon and Schuster, 1982.

Chomsky, Noam. *Problems of Knowledge and Freedom: The Russell Lectures.* New York: Vintage Books, 1971.

Chomsky, Noam. *Language and Mind.* New York: Harcourt Brace Jovanovich, 1972.

Christensen, Francis, and Bonnijean Christensen. *Notes Toward a New Rhetoric.* New York: Harper & Row, 1978.

Costello, William P. Lectures in "Linguistic Development and Applied Psycholinguistics." San Francisco State University, 1981–84.

Costello, William P. Lectures in "Psycholinguistics." San Francisco State University, 1982.

Crystal, David. *Profiling Linguistic Disability*. London: Edward Arnold Publishers, 1982.

Crystal, David, and Randolph Quirk. *Systems of Prosodic and Paralinguistic Features in English*. London: Mouton and Company, 1964.

Elgin, Suzette Haden. *The Gentle Art of Verbal Self-Defense*. New York: Dorset Press, 1980.

Fishman, J. A. "The Sociology of Language." In *Language and Social Context*, edited by Pier Paolo Gigliolo. Middlesex, England: Penguin Books, 1972.

Goldberger, Leo, and Shlomo Breznitz, eds. *Handbook of Stress: Theoretical and Clinical Aspects*. New York: The Free Press, 1982.

Goody, Ester N. "Towards a Theory of Questions." In *Questions and Politeness: Strategies in Social Interaction*, edited by Ester N. Goody. London: Cambridge University Press, 1978.

Gumperz, John. "The Speech Community." In *Language and Social Context*, edited by Pier Paolo Gigliolo. Middlesex, England: Penguin Books, 1972.

Howards, Melvin. *Reading Diagnosis and Instruction: An Integrated Approach*. Reston, Va.: Reston Publishing Company, 1980.

Jacobs, Roderick A., and Peter S. Rosenbaum. *Transformations, Style, and Meaning*. New York: John Wiley and Sons, 1971.

Lakoff, George, and Mark Johnson. *Metaphors We Live By*. Chicago. University of Chicago Press, 1980.

Lyons, John. *Semantics: Volumes I and II*. Cambridge: Cambridge University Press, 1977.

Martin, Judith. *Miss Manners' Guide to Excruciatingly Correct Behavior*. New York: Warner Books, 1982.

Mackay, Ian. *Introducing Practical Phonetics*. Boston: Little, Brown and Company, 1978.

Paulk, Walter. *How to Study in College*. Boston: Houghton Mifflin Company, 1984.

Piaget, Jean. *The Construction of Reality and the Child*. New York: Ballantine Books, 1954.

Piaget, Jean. *The Child's Conception of the World*. Lanham, Md.: Littlefield, Adams and Company, 1969.

Piaget, Jean. *The Child and Reality: Problems of Genetic Psychology*. Middlesex, England: Penguin Books, 1976.

Piaget, Jean. *Behavior and Evolution*. New York: Pantheon Books, 1978.

Robinson, William S. *Writing the Sentence: A Grammar for Teachers*. San Francisco: San Francisco State University, 1983.

Robinson, William S. Lectures in "Composition." San Francisco State University, 1981–83.

Scheglorr, E. A. "Notes on a Conversational Practice. Formulating Place." In *Language and Social Context,* edited by Pier Paolo Gigliolo. Middlesex, England: Penguin Books, 1972.

Searle, John. "What is a Speech Act?" In *Language and Social Context,* edited by Pier Paolo Gigliolo. Middlesex, England: Penguin Books, 1972.

Shaughnessy, Mina P. *Errors and Expectations: A Guide for the Teacher of Basic Writing.* New York: Oxford University Press, 1977.

Smith, Frank. *Understanding Reading.* New York: Holt, Rinehart, and Winston, 1971.

Smith, Frank. *Reading Without Nonsense.* New York: Teachers College Press, 1978.

Soames, Scott, and David M. Perlmutter. *Syntactic Argumentation and the Structure of English.* Berkeley: University of California Press, 1979.

Vygotsky, Lev S. *Thought and Language.* Cambridge, Mass.: MIT Press, 1962.

INDEX

Kay Thomsett is a writer/editor in the Department of Veterans Affairs in Washington, D.C.

Eve Nickerson is a retired secondary school teacher living in Portland, Oregon.